The Chocolate Therapist™

A User's Guide to the Extraordinary Health Benefits of Chocolate

Julie Pech

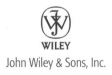

WILEY

John Wiley & Sons, Inc.

Published by John Wiley & Sons, Inc., Hoboken, New Jersey
Published simultaneously in Canada

Design by Forty-Five Degree Design LLC

Chart on page 173 reprinted by permission of Blommer Chocolate, 2009.

The information contained in this book is not intended to serve as a replacement for professional medical advice. Any use of the information in this book is at the reader's discretion. The author and the publisher specifically disclaim any and all liability arising directly or indirectly from the use or application of any information contained in this book. A health care professional should be consulted regarding your specific situation.

For general information about our other products and services, please contact our Customer Care Department within the United States at (800) 762-2974, outside the United States at (317) 572-3993 or fax (317) 572-4002.

Wiley also publishes its books in a variety of electronic formats. Some content that appears in print may not be available in electronic books. For more information about Wiley products, visit our web site at www.wiley.com.

Library of Congress Cataloging-in-Publication Data:
Pech, Julie.
   The chocolate therapist : a user's guide to the extraordinary health benefits of chocolate / Julie Pech.
      p. cm.
   Includes bibliographical references and index.
   ISBN 978-0-470-61351-1 (pbk.); ISBN 978-0-470-64292-4 (ebk.);
ISBN 978-0-470-64293-1 (ebk.); ISBN 978-0-470-64294-8 (ebk.)
   1.   Chocolate—Health aspects. 2.   Cookery (Chocolate) I.   Title.
   QP144.C46P43 2010
   613.2'8—dc22

                                                            2010006816

Printed in the United States of America

10 9 8 7 6 5 4 3 2 1

There are two types of people in the world—those who love chocolate and those who will soon. Perhaps this is why philosophers originally coined the phrase "we are all one." Once you understand the concept, life becomes considerably easier.

I dedicate this book to you: the chocolate lovers of the world.

Warning: Do not attempt to read this book without a dark chocolate bar in hand.

Contents

Acknowledgments

A special thank-you to my beautiful children, Britt and Blake, who endured years of product testing and research. They were unconditionally supportive of my efforts, repeatedly requesting more chocolate-based experiments to make certain we had everything right. Most important, they reminded me time and again to apply to myself what I always tell them: Hold on to your dreams until they come true.

Thank you to my friend and fellow author P. J. Campbell for helping me see that "serendipity happens" when we take time for ourselves. Her book *101 Author Tips* continues to be instrumental in my success. I'd also like to thank Rose Potts of Blommer Chocolate Company and Ann Noble for allowing me to publish their chocolate flavor and wine aroma wheels, respectively, in this book.

Thank you, Scott, for listening without advising and for thousands of unconditional hugs. And thank you to my lifelong friends DeEtte and Daryl for being there through everything else along the way.

I'm finally beginning to understand Lawrence Kushner's magical words "Everyone carries with them at least one piece to someone else's puzzle." God bless each of you.

Introduction

A FEW SHORT DECADES AGO smoking was harmless and cool, drinking a glass of red wine a day was the sign of a problem drinker, and eating bread and carbohydrates was the best way to lose weight. Even chocolate was considered bad for you. Fortunately, those days are behind us. We now know that smoking causes cancer, a daily glass of red wine is good for your heart, and one of the best ways to lose weight is by following a reduced-carbohydrate diet. Yet the most exciting news is that *chocolate* and *healthy* can finally be used in the same sentence. The Age of Chocolate has arrived.

With research results still coming in, many people are wondering how chocolate, a food on the "diet-don't" list for years, can be healthy. Yet surprisingly, chocolate has a variety of benefits for the body, such as mood-lifting neurotransmitters and powerful antioxidants. Chocolate also contains a healthy supply of vitamins and minerals and even stimulates the brain into releasing endorphins. In fact, once you've finished reading this book, you'll discover that it's possible to eat a little chocolate every day, guilt-free *and* without gaining weight. Admittedly, this statement seems too good to be true. I doubted it myself until a simple event triggered a full-scale investigation.

While deleting a collection of e-mail ads for bedroom stimulants, weight-loss pills, and guaranteed depression cures, I came across a single intriguing message titled "Why Chocolate Is Good for You." When I opened it, I discovered the following interesting facts: (1) Chocolate has more antioxidants by weight than red wine. (2) Chocolate releases endorphins in the brain that have been proved to uplift moods and reduce the sensation of pain. (3) Chocolate contains more than four hundred flavor compounds and plant chemicals, many of which benefit the body in some way.

The list went on, and the news got better with every sentence. As I surveyed my computer screen more closely, I realized that the e-mail for chocolate had arrived directly between the advertisements of our most pressing health issues. Having reviewed the informative essentials, I pondered, Wouldn't it be convenient if chocolate could solve our health problems?

All of this happened a few years ago, back when I had a career but had always longed to chase my capricious creative heart. I'd entertained the idea of writing a book for quite some time, and I wanted to write on a subject I felt passionate about. I'd spent most of my life studying nutrition in one form or another. I was a competitive athlete in my youth, which required paying constant attention to a diet that would help me perform at my personal best. My father was a nutritionist; I studied nutrition in college and spent much of my reading time poring over the latest diet books.

In fact, at any given time during my life, you'd more likely find me reading a diet or nutrition book as opposed to the latest best seller. I tried many of the diets, sometimes to lose weight and other times just to see how they affected the body. In what might have been a bit of a contradiction, a consuming passion for chocolate was never more than a wrapper away. The moment I read the "Why Chocolate Is Good for You" e-mail I knew my nutritional ship had come in. I sold my small corporate apparel company and set about researching how the loves of my life—nutrition and chocolate—intersected.

Yet when I began in 2004, high-quality research on chocolate was difficult to come by. Most of the chocolate-for-health news still consisted of rumors, and people laughed at the idea that they could actually have chocolate along with their daily glass of red wine. I didn't have a single contact in the chocolate industry before I began, but I wasn't about to let this minor detail stand in my way. I started firing off e-mails to anyone who looked like he or she might be able to help.

Within a few weeks the most amazing events occurred. I made connection after unexpected connection. People I'd never met referred me to universities, researchers, and scientists who were studying chocolate. Over time, I ended up with stacks of research that wasn't yet available to the public. So many coincidental events occurred time and again that I knew I was on the right path. Apparently, the "leap of faith" concept was the key—I had to take action before I could find who was out there to help. At parties the mere mention of the word *chocolate* prompted a swirl of highly intriguing conversations. Whenever I purchased stacks of chocolate bars at the checkout stand, curious strangers in line poured forth elixirlike tales of chocolate. Numerous friends leaped in with personal stories about how they used chocolate to self-medicate. Information on the health benefits of chocolate came my way, day after day. And, of course, everyone I talked to wanted to hear the facts so that they could embrace the concept of healthy chocolate enjoyment.

I decided to investigate other foods commonly added to chocolate bars as well, so my research expanded. I studied nuts, dried fruits and berries, flavored oils, and spices such as coffee, cinnamon, cayenne pepper, and mint. This new information revealed additional encouraging facts about food and health, all pointing to the obvious notion that eating real rather than processed foods has significant health benefits.

Some people may not define the chocolate bar as an unprocessed food. Yet once I'd considered the research, I discovered that it's possible to eat chocolate in a form that's quite close to the original cocoa bean. Because the cocoa bean is actually a fruit, eating chocolate provides many of the same benefits as eating fruit. The key is to eat the "right" kind of chocolate, so I focused on this area as well.

Ultimately, I uncovered the intricate details about chocolate that you'll learn while reading this book—why darker is better, how to read the labels to get the best chocolate, where to find good-quality chocolate, exactly which components of chocolate benefit health, how the industry is changing, and why spending a little more at the grocery store means saving money at your doctor's office. *The Chocolate Therapist* is divided into easy-to-follow chapters so that you can quickly absorb the facts and move directly to the chocolate remedies:

- "The Condensed History of Chocolate": Unique and entertaining facts that you can discuss at any social gathering.

- "From Cacao Tree to Chocolate Bar": A summary of cacao trees and the production process from bean to bar.

- "Healthy Investigation": An overview of the extraordinary health benefits of chocolate.

- "Selecting the Proper Chocolate": Learn how to choose the best chocolate for optimal health, how to read labels, what to look for, and what to avoid. Become an expert in your field.

- "Proper Chocolate Consumption": Quickly acquire the tasting skills of a distinguished chocolate connoisseur.

- "Chocolate Remedies": Exactly how and why chocolate can help alleviate an assortment of health issues.

After you finish the enticing chocolate center of the book, press on for even more entertainment in "Where Do You Hide Your Chocolate?" and "Chocolate and Wine Pairing" before you finish off with some delectable recipes. And there's no need to stop researching once you've finished the book. More studies than ever before are currently being conducted, all of them devoted to discovering chocolate's many hidden health benefits.

Remember Sir Francis Bacon's visionary words "Knowledge is power," a concept I can confirm as truth through personal experience. Who would have guessed that knowing so much about chocolate could lead to such an entertaining life? I have continuous projects in action, including a promising personal investigation: I've recommended to my children that they eat dark chocolate instead of other treats. As I hypothesized, they're taking to the idea rather well.

As another project, whenever I give in to the dessert tray, I now opt for a dark chocolate selection. In the past I mulled over every possible dessert. Now I simply decide which *chocolate* delicacy to enjoy. In the event that there are more than two, it's easy to convince someone else at the table to order one, while I select the other. Between the two of us, we're able to maximize the research potential.

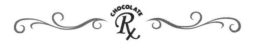

One

The Condensed History of Chocolate

HE HISTORY OF CHOCOLATE is ambiguous and full of mystery. Dates, places, and names conflict. Stories vary from one history book to the next. The people I met with to get to the bottom of the alleged facts seemed amused by my confusion. Apparently, if anyone genuinely believes that he or she understands the history of chocolate, that individual hasn't thoroughly researched the subject. It was true—the deeper I dug, the more controversy I found. Fortunately, I uncovered a moderately discernible path that I could count on.

Cocoa has been around for thousands of years, but it was the Maya who left the clearest documented record of its use, more than fifteen hundred years ago. Their elaborate system of hieroglyphics identifies the cocoa bean as one of their most esteemed and valuable articles of trade. Cocoa beans served as tribute to rulers and priests. The beans were buried in king's tombs and used in religious and matrimonial ceremonies. Maya texts also show that chocolate was consumed in a drink flavored with chili peppers and the dried flowers of a native plant.

As the Maya civilization collapsed, the Aztec empire rose to power. Like the Maya, the Aztecs embraced many of the symbolic rituals of chocolate, using it for their noble leaders and in honored religious ceremonies. It played a role in baptisms and marriage ceremonies, to the extent that five cocoa beans were exchanged between bride and groom as a pledge in the acceptance of marriage. Even to this day it's rumored that a man accepting a cup of specially prepared cocoa from the parents of a Bri Bri daughter in northern Costa Rica is offering a promise of marriage.

The fabled Aztec ruler Montezuma reportedly took goblets of the drink before attending to his harem, giving cocoa its much touted reputation as an aphrodisiac. It was regularly offered to the Aztec god Quetzalcoatl in ceremonies. In fact, cocoa's extraordinarily revered position within the Aztec and Maya civilizations prompted the Swedish naturalist Linnaeus to officially name the cacao tree *Theobroma Cacao* in 1753. *Theobroma* is Greek for "divine smell," but as years passed, *Theobroma Cacao* has come to be translated as "Food of the Gods."

Both the Maya and the Aztecs used cocoa beans as currency, lending credence to the phrase many of us heard as children, "Do you think money grows on trees?" Now you know that at one time it did. Ancient documents from the sixteenth century show that a tamale could be purchased for one cocoa bean, a rabbit for thirty beans, and a slave for a hundred beans. Even

Montezuma's treasure vaults were filled with cocoa beans instead of gold, much to the dismay of the gold-seeking Spaniards. The most coveted land in warfare was where cacao trees were most plentiful, because that land would continuously produce financial gains. Since drinking cocoa was literally "consuming money," chocolate was reserved for Aztec nobility. The commoners simply could not afford the luxury of eating money.

Christopher Columbus first laid eyes on the cocoa bean in 1502, and he's occasionally credited with introducing it to Spain. It's rumored that the tiny bean was overshadowed by the vast collection of larger treasures he returned with at the same time. Although it's true that Columbus may have been the first European to see the bean, he was not the first person to bring it to Spain.

The True History of Chocolate by Sophie and Michael Coe reports this interesting story. According to the journal of Columbus's son Ferdinand, in 1502 Columbus and his men encountered a huge Maya trading canoe filled with Indian slaves and goods from the Yucatán Peninsula. Columbus and his men captured the canoe and its treasures of fine cotton, war clubs with razorlike blades, small axes, and "almonds" (cocoa beans).

From his father's journals, Ferdinand translated that when "an almond fell, they [the natives] all stooped to pick it up, as if an eye had fallen." Lacking a translator, Columbus was not able to ascertain the value of the "almonds." After that encounter Columbus sailed on to what is now known as western Panama, where he discovered the gold he had been looking for. Four years later he died in Spain.

Conflicting reports make it difficult to determine exactly how chocolate was introduced to Europe, but it most certainly arrived in Spain before it did in any other country. Many history books report that Cortez brought the cocoa bean from the New World in 1519, nearly two decades after Columbus had his first encounter

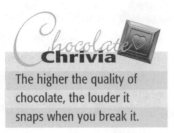

Chocolate Chrivia

The higher the quality of chocolate, the louder it snaps when you break it.

with it. Yet according to *The True History of Chocolate*, historical documentation of the contents of Cortez's ship bears no reference to cocoa at all.

Other accounts credit Cortez at a later date, in 1528, when he returned to Spain from the New World for a second time. This time he came back with a ship full of vast treasures: gold, silver, noblemen of Mexico, jaguars, an armadillo, and a bounty of other wonders. Some books say that Cortez introduced cocoa to Europe at this time, and others do not.

A different theory states that cocoa arrived in Europe by way of friars who had befriended the Kekchi Maya of Guatemala. Rather than conquer these rebellious Maya, a group of Dominican friars led by Bartolomé de las Casas made peace with the Kekchi. Based on documentation of that era, these successful efforts ultimately resulted in cocoa being brought to Europe.

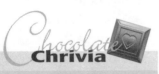

Chocolate Chrivia

Dark chocolate can be stored for up to a year in a cool, dry place (such as a wine cellar). White and milk chocolate can be stored for about six months.

In 1544, the friars brought a group of Kekchi Maya nobles to visit Prince Philip in Spain. Cocoa was among the many gifts they proffered. All historical references agree that from the mid-1500s on, the Spanish court enthusiastically adopted the custom of drinking chocolate. It became the preferred beverage of Spanish nobility. Each family developed its own special recipes, many of which can still be found today. Chocolate beverages were consumed in Spain almost exclusively for nearly a century, but controversy surrounds this notion as well.

While the Spaniards enjoyed their alleged "secret" use of chocolate, the Jesuit priests, convents, and monasteries had already begun to exploit the financial opportunities of cocoa. Founded by the Spaniard Ignatius Loyola in 1534, the Jesuit order was dedicated to strengthening the Catholic Church. By 1624, there were more than sixteen thousand Jesuit priests operating as a politically powerful group in Spain and the New World colonies.

Although the order worked for the church, it was rumored that its members regarded themselves as independent from both Spain and the New World. They built a strong and steadfast loyalty, and it didn't take long for them to discover that the cocoa business was extremely lucrative. The order's power and influence had a significant effect on the distribution of cocoa.

Regardless of *who* actually introduced cocoa to Spain, Cortez and his men were clearly instrumental in the process. They had been drinking cocoa in the New World for years by the time it arrived in Europe. And although they were impressed with the bean's value in the New World, they weren't exactly thrilled with its taste.

In fact, most of the Spanish invaders were initially repulsed by the drink. The Aztecs reportedly drank it cold and unsweetened. It was served with a frothy top that was whipped up by pouring the chocolate back and forth from containers held high over each other. The natives also added vanilla, chili pepper, and the dried flower petals of a local plant.

This approach created a bitter drink, far removed from the sugar-craving Spanish palate. Yet the lines between the Spanish invaders and Aztec tradition blurred during the next decade, when the Spaniards transformed the drink to suit their tastes. It first came to be served hot, rather than cold, followed by the addition of sweetened cane sugar. Spices such as cinnamon, aniseed, and black pepper helped complete the makeover.

Between the late 1500s and the mid-1600s, the custom of drinking chocolate spread from Spain to the rest of Europe. By the mid-1600s, chocolate houses had sprung up throughout the countryside. By the 1700s, chocolate was the preferred drink of wealthy Europeans, following the same elitist path that it had with the Maya, the Aztecs, and the Spaniards.

Doctors recommended it to cure ailments of all kinds, including insomnia and stomach disorders, and to strengthen and restore decaying health. People touted its use for everything positive, whether or not there was any justification at all. If you review historical journals regarding the medicinal uses of chocolate, keep in mind that much of the time, it was prescribed without the benefit of medical research to back up the claims.

Up until the 1820s, chocolate was consumed almost exclusively as a drink. But in 1828, the Dutchman Coenraad van Houten invented a hydraulic press that could compress the beans, causing the cocoa solids to separate from the cocoa butter. Freed from its 54 percent fat content, cocoa dried in a "cakelike" form. From this state, it could be pulverized for easy use in both drinks and solid confections. Large-scale production of chocolate followed shortly afterward.

The history of chocolate in Europe is long and eventful. Enthusiasts who wish to expand their knowledge of chocolate are advised to consult the previously mentioned reference *The True History of Chocolate*, a thorough account of humanity's adventures with chocolate.

Chocolate was first introduced to the United States in 1765, when cocoa beans were brought from the West Indies to Dorchester, Massachusetts. The John Hannon Company is credited with producing the first chocolate in the United States, marketed primarily for medicinal purposes. Hannon teamed up with Dr. James Baker to form the company, but when John Hannon was lost at sea, the name was changed to the Walter

Baker Company. The Baker Company still produces chocolate today, and many people don't realize that Baker's chocolate is so named for the man. It's a convenient coincidence that this same chocolate is typically used for baking.

It took more than a century for chocolate to establish a notable presence in the United States. In 1894, a young man by the name of Milton Hershey founded what has become one of the largest U.S. chocolate companies, the Hershey Chocolate Company.

Milton Hershey was a tenacious man, attempting and subsequently failing no less than three times to start a candy manufacturing company. He found his initial success in making caramels, and the English were his biggest customers. On a trip abroad, however, he discovered that the British were cutting his caramels down and covering them with chocolate. After he witnessed children chewing the chocolate off the caramels and spitting the rest out, chocolate became his new direction.

Hershey sold the caramel business to focus wholly on chocolate. Eager to expand into the potential chocolate market, he searched for a unique and appealing approach. Daniel Peter had recently invented evaporated milk, and Henri Nestlé had applied it to a chocolate recipe. After some experimenting of his own, Hershey discovered that this new, lighter version of the original treat was immensely popular with consumers because of its mild and creamy taste. When the Hershey's milk chocolate bar was introduced in 1900, a new era in chocolate began.

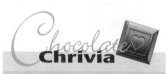

Chocolate Chrivia

Napoléon reportedly carried chocolate with him on a regular basis, eating it whenever he needed quick energy.

Within a relatively short period of time, Hershey revolutionized chocolate production. Not only was he manufacturing a chocolate that appealed to nearly everyone's taste, but he began to mass-produce it in a variety of products, such as bars and wafers. By doing this, he effectively lowered the price and made it available to people of all income levels. The future was eminent: chocolate was well on its way to becoming one of the country's most popular snacks.

Today the average American consumes approximately twelve pounds of chocolate per year. Although that may sound like a mountain of chocolate, it averages out to one pound of chocolate per month, or one candy bar every three days. After some careful calculating, you may realize that you've been consuming more than your fair share of the quota. If so, you could be drawing from your international heritage. The list on this page shows a few of the world's more dedicated chocolate-consuming countries.

As evidenced by recent articles with titles such as "Chocolate: The New Health Food" and "Chocolate Healing," there's never

Country	Lb/Yr per Person
Switzerland	23*
United Kingdom	22
Germany	20
Belgium	19
Norway	19
Austria	16
Ireland	16
Australia	13

Source: Caobisco, www.caobisco.com.

*The astute statistical observer will note that Switzerland's extraordinary per/person consumption rate probably does not account for the fact that a good portion of its chocolate is purchased by tourists. Thus, the Swiss likely consume smaller amounts than reported. But those English!

been a better time to restock your cupboards with chocolate. I suspect that at some point, chocolate will be added to the new food pyramid, right next to its culinary cousins, the fruits. After all, chocolate is good for you. The key, of course, is to educate yourself about which chocolate to eat for health, how much to eat, what to look for on the labels, and what to stay away from. So, off to school you go.

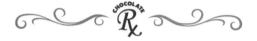

Two

From Cacao Tree to Chocolate Bar

C HOCOLATE'S AMAZING HEALTH benefits stem from the fact that it's made from the ground-up seeds of a fruit tree. Seeds are the most nutrient-dense and antioxidant-rich part of a plant. The following cacao-tree-to-chocolate-bar description will give you a working knowledge of chocolate that few people have at present, thus providing an excellent opportunity for you to display your chocolate finesse at social gatherings.

The Cacao Tree and Where It Grows

Chocolate starts its journey on the *Theobroma Cacao* tree, a finicky plant that grows only in a narrow band that stretches 20 degrees north and south of the equator. It requires a very hot, humid environment to flourish. Slightly more than thirty countries in the world (listed below) are estimated to be able to grow cacao.

Africa: Madagascar, Ivory Coast, Ghana, São Tomé, Nigeria, Sierra Leone, Toga, Equatorial Guinea, Congo, Sri Lanka

Asia: Malaysia, Indonesia, Philippines, Papua New Guinea

Caribbean: Grenada, Haiti, Jamaica, Trinidad, Cuba, Dominican Republic, Tobago

Central and South America: Brazil, Ecuador, Colombia, Venezuela, Mexico, Costa Rica, Panama, Peru, Bolivia

South Pacific: Java, Fiji, West Samoa, Hawaii (United States)

Cacao trees reach a height of approximately twenty-five feet and need plenty of shade and moisture to grow properly. To help accomplish this, farmers typically plant taller trees such as banana, papaya, macadamia nut, and mango near cacao trees. Partially cleared forests also make ideal settings for the high-maintenance cacao trees. Despite all of this pampering, in any given year, 50 to 75 percent of the world's crop can be destroyed by disease or natural causes, making cocoa a fairly volatile crop.

There are three primary types of trees:

1. **Criollo**: This is the original wild cacao tree, considered by many to have the best-tasting beans. Because of this, devout chocolate connoisseurs and artisans spend considerable time tracking the perfect Criollo trees. Once they find them, they may contract to buy the farmer's crop for years, thereby assuring a continued supply.

The pods produced by the Criollo tree are soft, and the beans are typically purple or pale purple in color. Flavors vary from tree to tree and country to country, but many people in the industry consider Ecuador to be one of the best producers of proprietary beans. Because the Criollo is prone to disease and natural destruction, there are fewer of this type of tree than of any other breed in the world. Estimates of the number of Criollo trees range from .1 to 1 percent of the world's total cacao trees.

2. **Forastero**: This is the hardiest breed of cacao tree. The Forastero produces beans with bold and strong flavors. The most popular Forastero is the Amelonado, grown primarily in West Africa and Brazil. The pod is smooth and yields anywhere from thirty to forty lavender to purple beans. Forastero trees make up approximately 90 percent of the world's cacao trees.

3. **Trinitario**: The Trinitario derives its name from Trinidad, the isle of its origin. It is a hybrid of the Criollo and Forastero trees. Beans from the Trinitario tree have inherited the more refined and unique flavors of the Criollo but also the hardiness of the Forastero tree—an ideal combination that offers the best of both worlds.

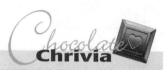

Chocolate Chrivia

A friend of mine who trades cocoa beans told me that during a recent trip to South America, he brought some chocolate with him for the cocoa farmer he buys beans from. The farmer had never tasted finished chocolate. He was surprised to learn that the chocolate my friend shared with him had been created from his beans.

This was a surprise to me—even countries that have been growing cacao for centuries have no idea what to do with it!

Unlike the Criollo, these trees are cultivated rather than wild. They're found primarily in the Caribbean, Cameroon, and Papua New Guinea and make up the remaining 9 percent of the world's cacao trees.

Transforming Cacao Pods into the Food of the Gods

The trees begin to bear foot-long pods when they're four to five years old. They sprout from every part of the tree, even the trunk. It's not a picturesque arrangement, nothing like a typical fruit dangling peacefully on the end of a branch. In fact, the growing pods have a very unique look—think football meets cactus. At first glance it hardly seems plausible that the chocolate we know and love is derived from this odd-shaped fruit. The process is so complex that once you know how it's done, it becomes obvious why it took people hundreds of years to use the homely plant to create the chocolate we eat today.

A single tree produces between twenty and thirty pods per year, and each pod produces approximately forty beans. That's a thousand to twelve hundred beans per tree per year. It takes approximately four hundred beans to make a pound of chocolate. After it's all added up, each tree produces only enough beans to make two pounds of chocolate per year.

When I crunched the numbers, I realized that as a two-ounce-a-day consumer, I'm running through the production of approximately twenty-five cocoa trees a year. At the time of this book's printing, cocoa production levels currently meet world demand. But when future consumption increases as people begin to eat more chocolate for health benefits, some cocoa-producing companies expect a shortage in the years to come.

At harvesttime the pods are hacked off the tree with a machete and split open. Inside the pods, cocoa beans (sometimes called seeds) grow packed in a sweet pulp, twenty to forty beans per pod, depending on the tree varietal. The entire mass of beans and pulp is scooped out of the shells and piled into heaps or boxes, which commences the first stage, called fermentation. The heat of the region's climate causes the sweet pulp to disintegrate into vinegar and alcohol, which drains away and leaves only the beans. Proper fermentation is so crucial to bringing out the flavors that many chocolate companies create strict guidelines on the process for farmers to follow. If the fermentation is done improperly, an entire crop can be ruined.

Fermentation is followed by a drying period. This process is also essential for flavor enhancement and can be very labor-intensive, often requiring as many as five to ten days to complete. Traditional methods involve sun-drying, where the beans are laid out on large cement platforms and allowed to dry in the sun. When it rains, they are covered to prevent mold and mildew and are uncovered again when the sun returns. Because it rains more than once a day in many regions, constant supervision is required during the drying process. In recent years, more advanced drying methods have been devised, making the process shorter.

Next, the beans go through a roasting process, another key step in flavor production. A very thin shell covers each bean. When the bean is heated, the cocoa butter in it expands, causing the shells to burst. The shells are winnowed away by a large blower, leaving broken bits of beans, commonly called nibs. Because they're literally the broken seeds of a fruit tree, the nibs are rich in vitamins, nutrients, protein, and antioxidants. They can be eaten whole as well. They're somewhat bitter and nutty, but it doesn't take long to acquire a taste for them, and many people find them quite enjoyable.

From this point, the nibs get rolled back and forth between large rollers. Because they're made up of approximately 54% cocoa butter and 46% cocoa solids, rolling and pressing turns them into a thick chocolate soup called chocolate liquor. There's no alcohol in this kind of liquor—just pure cocoa beans ground into a rich chocolate puree.

In the final step, additional pressing and grinding of the cocoa liquor causes it to separate into cocoa butter and cocoa solids. The solids are pressed into cakes, pulverized into cocoa powder, and used to make all things chocolate. The cocoa butter is of course used in the creation of chocolate, but some of it is also sold to the cosmetics industry.

Almost all of the health benefits of chocolate are in the cocoa powder, which is why dark chocolate is better for you. Liquids and fats have literally been squeezed out of the seeds, leaving only the cocoa solids—the richest and most potent part of the fruit.

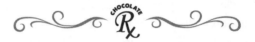

Three

Healthy Investigation

HOCOLATE CONTAINS an extraordinary collection of compounds known to benefit the body, but what we seem to hear most often is that it's "rich in antioxidants." Most people know they're supposed to eat antioxidants to promote good health. Yet while I was on a speaking tour, I discovered that many people have no idea exactly what antioxidants are, what they do in the body, where they come from, and why chocolate has so many of them. This chapter will help clear up the confusion.

Antioxidants are media darlings because of their extraordinary health-enhancing properties. They do what their name implies: "anti" and "oxidant," meaning they keep cells from oxidizing. Oxidation is the breakdown of healthy cells, and, obviously, if you want a healthy body, you want to minimize the destruction of healthy cells.

Any type of molecule can undergo an oxidation reaction, in which it loses an electron. The resulting molecule is called a free radical. There are different types of free radicals, but the type that concerns us in relation to health degeneration is the oxygen free radical. These molecules migrate through the bloodstream looking for electrons to rebalance their structure. They steal electrons from our healthy cells, and over time, this causes cells to degenerate. When the body breaks down, the root cause is free radicals. They're the primary cause of more than two hundred major illnesses, including cancer, heart disease, diabetes, arthritis, Alzheimer's disease, and many more.

All of the bad news about free radicals makes it obvious that the key to good health would simply be to avoid them. Unfortunately, it's not that easy because they're by-products of digestion, metabolism, and respiration. As we digest food, exercise, and breathe, free radicals are formed. So if you've alive, you're producing free radicals. The more active you are, the more you generate. Top athletes are at the greatest risk because they eat, metabolize, and breathe more than the rest of us do. Short of dying, there's no way to avoid free radicals.

Fortunately, the body has its own natural defense system, but the highly contaminated environment we live in today often overwhelms the body's ability to do the job on its own. Free radicals are also created when we breathe in air pollution, eat processed and greasy foods, use artificial sweeteners, stay out in the sun, experience stress, smoke, drink alcohol, undergo medical X-rays, take various medications, use inexpensive skin-care products, and come in contact with thousands of other toxins. It's estimated that a single cell in the body can experience thousands of attacks per day from free radicals that try to break it down. The body needs extra help in fighting the repeated assaults, and this is where antioxidant-rich foods come in.

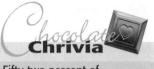

Chocolate Chrivia

Fifty-two percent of Americans claim chocolate as their favorite flavor. Vanilla and berry flavors tie for second.

Antioxidants

Antioxidants rid the body of free radicals in two ways—either by donating one of their own electrons to neutralize the free radical or by grabbing onto it and pulling it out of the body. By nature, antioxidants consist of rings of single and double bonds, but a single bond is all they need to stay together. They can rearrange their double bonds to grab a destructively charged free radical as it passes and then drag it out of the body. Antioxidants even have the ability to start chain reactions of activity that neutralize many free radicals.

The main antioxidants are vitamins A, C, and E; coenzyme Q10 (CoQ10); alpha lipoic acid; and selenium. They come primarily from fresh fruits and vegetables, and, of course, you can take them as supplements. There are also considerable antioxidants in green tea and red wine. But the good news for chocolate lovers is that out of all of the possible food choices, chocolate has one of the highest levels of antioxidants per gram of any food measured to date.

The reason chocolate is so highly rated on the antioxidant chart is that it's made from the ground-up seeds of a fruit tree. As was mentioned in chapter 2, the process starts with the fruit: its seeds are extracted, liquids and fats are removed, and the finished product is pressed into cocoa cakes. So chocolate is made from the essence of the cacao plant—the seeds. This is why it compares in antioxidant value to many fruits (see the ORAC [oxygen radical absorbance capacity] chart below).

ORAC of Certain Foods	
Food	**Units per 100 Grams**
Undutched cocoa powder	34,396
Acai berries	18,500
Dark chocolate	13,120
Milk chocolate	6,740
Prunes	5,770
Red wine (3.5 oz)	3,524
Pomegranate	3,307
Raisins	2,830
Blueberries	2,400
Blackberries	2,035
Kale	1,770
Cranberries	1,750
Strawberries	1,540
Spinach	1,260
Raspberries	1,220
Brussels sprouts	980
Plums	949
Alfalfa sprouts	930
Broccoli florets	890
Oranges	750
Red grapes	739
Red bell pepper	710

| Cherries | 670 |
| Kiwi | 610 |

Source: U.S. Department of Agriculture, 2007.

When you eat 100 grams of each of these foods, the ORAC score listed here measures the free radicals that are neutralized on consumption. Antioxidants neutralize free radicals in the body—think of them as being like toxin vacuum cleaners. The more foods you eat that are high in antioxidants, the healthier you will be. Of course, you wouldn't eat 100 grams of dark chocolate a day (this chart is based on 70% dark chocolate), but even if you cut the quantity by 75 percent and ate only 25 grams, you'd still be at 3,280 on the ORAC chart, much higher than most foods at the 100-gram level.

Red wine is highly touted for its antioxidant value, but eating a dark chocolate bar provides twice the antioxidant benefit as drinking a glass of red wine. Like chocolate, red wine is also made by pressing the seeds of a fruit. But wine still contains a substantial amount of liquid, whereas chocolate does not, which is why chocolate is higher in antioxidant value by weight than red wine is.

Another unique characteristic of chocolate is that its antioxidants are readily absorbed by the body, so you don't have to consume vast quantities to obtain significant results. According to research conducted at Cornell University, even a very small amount of commercial-grade chocolate provides benefits to the body. Another report showed that only one ounce of chocolate, or about half of a regular-size candy bar, causes a measurable increase in antioxidants in the body. This study was done using an average chocolate bar. One that has a higher percentage of cocoa would be even more beneficial.

To get really serious about incorporating more antioxidants into your diet, add unsweetened cocoa powder to some of your recipes. It contains more than two times the amount

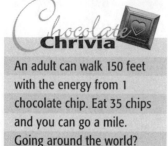

of antioxidants that standard 70% dark chocolate has, or 34,000 on the ORAC chart. Although you might not want to add cocoa powder to your morning coffee, take a look at the collection of excellent dark chocolate recipes in chapter 9. You'll find that they help make the transition easy.

Vitamins, Minerals, Fiber, and Protein

Dark chocolate also contains minerals, vitamins, fiber, and protein. Its most prevalent minerals are magnesium, copper, potassium, and calcium. Magnesium is used for protein synthesis, energy production, nerve impulse transmission, and muscle relaxation. A 1.75-gram bar of milk chocolate provides 8 percent of the daily magnesium requirement, while a serving of dark chocolate can provide as much as 15 percent.

Copper is used in the body to synthesize collagen and neurotransmitters. Copper deficiencies have been connected to cardiovascular abnormalities, particularly later in life. A typical milk chocolate bar contains approximately 19 percent of the recommended daily requirement for copper, but a dark chocolate bar contains approximately 34 percent. A University of Nebraska study discovered not only that most Americans are copper deficient but also that chocolate can contribute up to 22 percent of their daily copper intake.

There is also some fiber in chocolate, although it's a relatively small amount. A 3.5-ounce bar of 70% dark chocolate contains approximately 5 grams of fiber. The recommended daily allowance for fiber is 25 grams for women and 38 grams for men, so a good-size bar can provide as much as 20 percent of your recommended fiber. But you'd be far over the healthy one-ounce limit if you ate the whole bar. Yet it's possible to get more fiber from chocolate by eating it in its pure form—either whole beans or nibs. They're kind of bitter, but the fiber hasn't been processed out.

Chocolate even has a little protein, which makes sense, considering that it's made from seeds. All seeds contain high percentages of protein because protein is the building block of life, and seeds are the starting point. Processing removes some of it, but most good-quality 70% dark chocolate bars still report a protein content of about 4 grams per serving. Just like the fiber, eat whole cocoa beans or cocoa nibs to get more protein from chocolate.

Fats in Chocolate: Good or Bad?

Chocolate has taken the rap for being a high-fat, cholesterol-raising enemy in the diet war for good reason: most chocolate does, in fact, contain large amounts of harmful fats and sugar. Yet you can educate yourself to choose healthy forms of chocolate once you learn a little about the fat it contains.

There are primarily three types of fat in chocolate: 35–41 percent oleic acid, 34–39 percent stearic acid, and 23–30 percent palmitic acid. Linoleic acid rounds out the total at 5 percent. Oleic acid is considered a healthy fat because it actually helps lower cholesterol levels. It's the same fat that is found in other fruits, such as olives and avocados, which is not surprising because chocolate is made from a fruit.

Stearic acid is a saturated fat, but it is cholesterol-neutral and does not cause cholesterol levels to rise. A number of studies have shown that stearic acid is not absorbed as other fats are and passes through the body up to twice as fast. The remaining metabolized stearic acid breaks down into oleic acid, the same healthy fat mentioned previously. Whenever you see "saturated" fat on the label of a chocolate bar that contains only cocoa butter, this primarily refers to the stearic acid fat content. But if the ingredient label includes butter fat, hydrogenated oil, or milk fat, you're looking at less healthy saturated fats.

The only "bad" fat in chocolate is palmitic acid, a saturated fat that has been determined to raise cholesterol. Yet because palmitic acid is only 25 percent of the total fat, its disadvantages are outweighed by the advantages of the three good fats. As noted later, in chapter 6, many studies have shown that when subjects eat cocoa butter, as opposed to regular butter, low-density lipoproteins (LDLs) are reduced and high-density lipoproteins (HDLs) are raised. This is exactly the type of cholesterol action your body and your doctor want to see.

The other remaining fat, linoleic acid, is an essential fatty acid that is extremely important to the body. Essential fatty acids (EFAs) are types of fat that the body is unable to synthesize and that must be obtained in the diet. Despite making up only 5 percent of the total fat in chocolate, linoleic acid plays a significant role in promoting good health. The weight-loss frenzy that led people to reduce fat in their diets has actually decreased the necessary good fats, as well as the unhealthy fats. The resulting problem is a deficiency in EFAs for as much as 60 percent of the population.

Many people run when they hear the word *fat*, yet without fats in our diet, we would wither up and die. Essential fatty acid deficiencies are only a small part of the problem as people seek to avoid every conceivable item that contains fat and replace it with a fat-free product. This strategy ends up accentuating food cravings and ensures perpetual hunger (see "Food Cravings" in chapter 6).

The body needs fat, so don't deprive yourself of all fats. Instead, educate yourself on which fats are necessary for your body to properly function, and make sure to include them in your diet. The brain is 60 percent fat. Hormone production and appetite control are regulated by fats. When fat is missing from the diet, these processes don't function

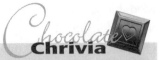

Chrivia

Chocolate can be lethal to dogs because they lack the enzyme to metabolize the theobromine contained in chocolate. Two ounces of chocolate can poison a ten-pound puppy.

well. Understanding fats will provide many additional benefits beyond a trimmer waistline. One of the world's foremost dietary experts is author Mary Enig. Her book *Know Your Fats* is an excellent resource for people looking for more information on this subject.

Conflicting Research?

To get a balanced perspective on the research, I studied the pros and cons of chocolate's health benefits and looked for conflicting data as well. A number of studies declared that the nutrient content of chocolate is so limited that it's insignificant, yet I discovered considerable research that had an opposing view. In fact, not only did the research disagree about the health benefits of chocolate; conflicting views predominated regarding what we should eat, particularly among top-selling diet-book authors.

Best-selling author Barry Sears (*The Zone: A Dietary Road Map to Lose Weight Permanently*) claims that if you have a healthy diet, almost all of your essential nutrients can come from your food. He supports this theory throughout the book by reminding us that considerable research has shown vitamin supplements to be of little use to the human body, because a large percentage of them end up being excreted.

Yet renowned authors Robert O. and Shelly Redford Young provide a long list of required supplements for ideal health in their popular book *The pH Miracle*. Many other authors agree with this strategy as well. These are merely two examples of how popular diet books often present diametrically opposed viewpoints. So, can we get everything we need from food or do we need supplements?

In his book *Diet for a New America*, Pulitzer Prize–nominated author John Robbins notes that within the last two hundred years, the United States has lost approximately 75 percent of its topsoil. Many other parts of the world have followed suit. Topsoil is where plants absorb minerals. Although fertilizing adds nitrogen, phosphorus, and potassium, it does not provide trace minerals. No matter how much we eat, we're still mineral-starved because most trace minerals no longer exist in our foods. The majority of diet professionals seem to believe that even perfect eating can't address all of our nutritional needs; we need supplements.

Perhaps the best strategy takes both views into consideration: a combination of supplements and nutrient-dense foods. Dark chocolate is an excellent food choice because it's so rich in nutrients. In addition, because cacao trees grow in the rich soils of the tropical rain forest, the trees can absorb more nutrients than the nutrient-starved agricultural produce that many of us consume today.

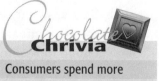

Chocolate Chrivia

Consumers spend more than $20 billion worldwide per year on chocolate.

Your Overall Eating Strategy

Cells replicate using substances contained in the foods you eat. A vitamin- and mineral-packed, antioxidant-rich food will help build more energetic and vibrant cells. Cooked, processed, stripped, and fried foods will merely cause the development of nutrient-starved cells. Compare the process to building a house—if you start with dead, dried-out trees and shrubs, you'll be homeless after the first strong wind. Build your house with strong, good-quality materials, and you'll have a place to stay for a while.

To get the most value from your chocolate, choose brands that have a high percentage of cocoa. If you're going to eat chocolate for health, you simply must eat the most nutritious types. After reading through the research, you'll be convinced of what you always hoped would be true: that chocolate is truly good for you.

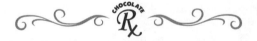

Four

Selecting the Proper Chocolate

THIS CHAPTER EXPLAINS the difference between good chocolate and bad, between heart health and heart disease, and between high cholesterol and low; it also covers weight gain versus weight loss. Choosing the proper chocolate is as important as selecting the right fuel for your car; if you get it wrong, you're not going anywhere, except maybe to a weight-loss seminar. A good percentage of the chocolate that's on the market is loaded with sugar and unhealthy fats. Rather than grabbing the nearest bar in sight, take time to learn a few simple concepts that will help you choose the best chocolate.

Just because the wrapper says "dark" doesn't mean it's healthy. Learning how to read ingredient labels is the key to knowing what to choose. Cocoa powder, cocoa, cocoa liquor, or some type of cocoa solids should be the first ingredient in the bar. Look for a brand that states the cocoa content on the wrapper, ideally a minimum of 60% dark or higher.

Brands that don't state the percentage of cocoa probably don't contain enough to make it worth revealing. Some of the mainstream brands contain less than 20% cocoa powder. When a chocolate bar contains only 20% cocoa, the remaining 80 percent of the bar is primarily sugar and fat. By selecting brands that list cocoa content, you keep sugar and fat intake to a reasonable minimum. You'll also get more nutrients and less sugar at the same time, the ultimate double positive.

Another reason to go dark is that adding dairy products (such as milk) to chocolate may adversely affect the body's ability to absorb chocolate's antioxidants. In a study done at the University of Glasgow in Scotland, researchers discovered that when volunteers were given milk chocolate or milk with their dark chocolate, there was no significant increase in blood antioxidant activity. Their recommendation was not to eat dairy products at the same time you eat chocolate.

Perhaps the most significant reason to go dark is that the antioxidants, vitamins, minerals, and protein are *all* in the cocoa powder. The darker the chocolate, the more value at every level. According to a report posted on the *Journal of Agricultural and Food Chemistry*'s Web site, there's a significant difference in antioxidant content from low-percentage cocoa to the highest. The study measured antioxidant and polyphenol content in six forms of chocolate: natural cocoa, unsweetened baking chocolate, dark chocolate, semisweet baking chips, milk chocolate, and chocolate syrup. The most significant factor in determining antioxidant content and activity was the percentage of nonfat cocoa solids.

Ice cream lovers: chocolate syrup might taste good, but it doesn't count in the "good for health" chocolate category.

Cocoa Percentages

To help you hone your chocolate-selection skills, I've listed the cocoa percentages as required by the U.S. government. You'd think it would be fairly basic, but federal regulations differ from country to country. The following list is based on a set of guidelines in the United States called the Standards of Identity. If the chocolate is in one of the following categories, it should contain the percentage described here. The rules in Europe are a little more stringent than in the United States.

Cocoa powder: Made by pulverizing defatted cocoa liquor. Nearly all of the cocoa butter has been removed. It's 100% pure cocoa powder.

Unsweetened chocolate: Called cocoa liquor and also known as bitter or baking chocolate; it consists of pure roasted and ground cocoa beans, containing both cocoa solids and cocoa butter, and has a very strong chocolate flavor.

Bittersweet chocolate: Cocoa liquor with added sugar and cocoa butter. Typically, 63–72% cocoa content listed on the bar, but the minimum requirement is only 35% cocoa liquor.

Dark chocolate: Cocoa liquor with added sugar and cocoa butter. Required minimums by law are 15% cocoa liquor in the United States and 35% cocoa solids in Europe. It's also called "sweet chocolate." For optimal health benefits, dark chocolate should contain 60% or more cocoa.

Semisweet chocolate: Dark chocolate with a higher sugar content, which is generally used for baking. Typically, it contains 52–62% cacao.

Milk chocolate: Chocolate liquor with cocoa butter, sugar, and milk products. It is required to contain 10% cocoa liquor in the United States and 25% cocoa solids in Europe. In the United States it must also contain 12% milk solids and a little more than 3% milk fat. It can be made with powdered or evaporated milk.

White chocolate: A confection made with cocoa butter, sugar, flavorings, and no cocoa solids. It should contain at least 20% cocoa butter to lawfully be termed white chocolate. It also typically contains as much as 14% milk solids and 3.5% milk fat.

White Chocolate Lovers Take Note

There are no antioxidants or health benefits in white chocolate. The antioxidants in chocolate come from the cocoa powder, and because the cocoa has been removed from white chocolate, the benefits are gone, too. The only reason it's called "white chocolate" is that it's made with cocoa butter. Make sure to read the labels, though, because many confections that pass as white chocolate don't even contain cocoa butter. They're merely knockoffs that were designed to look and taste like white chocolate.

Although the cocoa butter in white chocolate has not been shown to raise cholesterol levels, it won't reduce them either, because the cocoa has been removed. When you're eating chocolate for health, white chocolate shouldn't be part of the program. Enjoy it on special occasions, but choose dark for the daily plan.

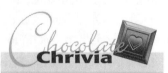
Chocolate Chrivia

Chocolate was consumed exclusively as a drink for many centuries. British chocolate maker J. S. Fry and Sons is credited with creating the first solid chocolate in 1830.

Wrapper Reading 101

Even if you've discovered a nice selection of 60%+ bars, there's a good chance you're still standing glassy-eyed in the chocolate aisle, thinking, How am I supposed to know which one to buy? Which ingredients are good? Which ones are bad? What should I look for? What about the order of ingredients? How much is too much? What does the percentage of cocoa mean? This one has saturated fats on the label—won't it give me high cholesterol? Almost all chocolate has sugar in it—isn't that bad for me?

In my presentations, I've heard these questions and more. People also ask me, "What is the best chocolate?" or "Which one is your favorite?" There really isn't a right answer because each person has a different palate and will enjoy different chocolates. This section of the book helps clear up the confusion and shows you how to find the great-quality, health-promoting chocolate that you love. Once you have a healthy piece of chocolate in hand, the next step is to compare it to a few other healthy chocolates to see which one you like best.

Yes, this is homework, but you'll get no mercy from me. I have to do this at least once a week and sometimes daily, so I know for a fact that it's just not that hard. To get on top of your "bar trek" in only a few minutes, use this nine-step how-to-read-the-wrappers guide.

1. **Chocolate:** As mentioned earlier, the first ingredient should be chocolate or some rendition of it, such as cocoa, cocoa beans, cocoa liquor (no alcohol here—simply pure cacao), cocoa solids, and cocoa mass. You're also looking for 60% or higher cocoa content. Once you start reading the labels, you'll notice "sugar" listed as the first ingredient in many popular dark chocolate brands, which, of course, is not ideal for health.

2. **Cocoa:** Look for nonalkali cocoa, or nondutched, although it's still somewhat unusual. Dutching darkens chocolate

and mellows its naturally acidic flavor, but, unfortunately, it also removes many of the antioxidants, as much as 25–75 percent, depending on processing. Nondutched isn't imperative, but it's something to keep in mind if you have a choice.

3. **Cocoa butter**: Cocoa butter should be the only fat in the bar. You may or may not see the words *cocoa butter* if *cocoa liquor* is written on the wrapper (it's part of the liquor), but you'll definitely see it when the ingredients list unsweetened cocoa or cocoa powder. Hydrogenated fats, animal fats, and vegetable oils are not necessary.

4. **Sugar**: The best sugars are organic or raw sugarcane, evaporated cane juice, beet sugar, plain sugar, and agave. Not as good are corn syrup, high fructose corn syrup, glucose, maltose, and other ingredients that end with *ose*.

5. **Soy lecithin**: Most bars contain this ingredient as an emulsifier—it helps chocolate maintain its form and consistency. A number of companies don't put soy lecithin in their bars, however, so it isn't absolutely necessary.

6. **Vanilla**: Look for vanilla beans, vanilla, or organic vanilla. Vanillin (with the *n* on the end) is an artificial flavoring, so look for the *a* on the end for the real deal.

7. **Sugar-free chocolates**: These are not recommended, because most sugar-free sweeteners are synthetic. Many contain aspartame, sucralose, saccharin, and maltitol—products that tend to upset the stomach and cause gas. Eating dark chocolate with nuts is healthier than eating sugar-free chocolate. The fat and protein in the nuts contribute to making a dark chocolate and nut bar only 33 on the glycemic index, thus raising blood sugar less than a handful of grapes does (read more about the glycemic

index in appendix B). Diabetics should look for evaporated cane juice or agave nectar, both of which are lower-glycemic sweeteners than processed sugar.

8. **Fair Trade:** This means that the manufacturer has paid a higher-than-market price for the cocoa beans to help support the indigenous farmers who grow it. This is always a good choice whenever it's available—invest in the future of the cocoa market.

9. **Organic:** This means no chemicals; the optimal situation for your body.

Remember that top-quality chocolate contains only four to five ingredients at most. Also, focus on pure chocolate bars with infusions such as nuts, spices, and dried fruits, as opposed to sugar-laden chocolates.

You might also consider reading the entire wrapper to expand your adventures in chocolate. Many companies provide details inside the wrappers about their start-up stories, values, sustainable growing programs, Fair Trade status, Rain Forest Alliance work, and much more. There's a history of chocolate on many wrappers, and really, what else are you studying these days? Why not make it chocolate? Some bars even offer love poems, making your one-stop gift all the more meaningful and heartfelt.

Organic Chocolate

Choosing organic is always a good idea. The first reason is obvious: when cocoa beans are grown free from chemicals and pesticides, these harmful additives won't be passed on to your body. But there's another reason to consider as well.

The recent demand for higher-quality chocolate has increased substantially. Unfortunately, this trend has caused cocoa growers (particularly on the Ivory Coast in Africa) to pay their workers wages far below poverty levels. Some of these growers also use young children as field laborers.

Organic chocolate, on the other hand, is less likely to be produced by companies that are responsible for these degrading labor situations. Because organic growers are able to charge more for their cocoa, they generally pay their workers higher wages and also refrain from using children as laborers.

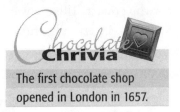

Chrivia

The first chocolate shop opened in London in 1657.

Fair Trade Chocolates

Fair Trade is also something to consider, as are chocolate companies that support the Rain Forest Alliance, farmers' co-ops, and other ecologically responsible organizations. Typically, companies have paid a higher-than-market price for their cocoa to help support the cocoa farmers. The Fair Trade mark also guarantees that children have not been forced into labor for production. Because an estimated 85 percent of the world's cocoa supply is grown by indigenous farmers, their well-being is imperative to the overall health of the cocoa market. Whenever you enjoy fine-quality chocolate, purchase brands that embrace social responsibility as well. After considering the options, you have plenty of good reasons to buy organic, Fair Trade, and Rain Forest Alliance brands. You'll get superior-quality chocolate, more antioxidants, and no pesticides, and you'll support the people who labor to bring you the delights you love.

When you consider the cost of a double latte, which is devoid of nutritional value, the cost of a vitamin-packed dark chocolate bar suddenly becomes a bit more reasonable. So, for the sake of your health, as well as of supporting a politically correct chocolate industry, take the plunge and invest in top-quality chocolate. There's no question that you'll have to pay a little more, but you're worth it. Otherwise, the money you *don't* spend on healthy choices will probably end up going to your health-care practitioner later.

Are Your Assorted Boxed Chocolate Days Over?

Filled chocolates are acceptable for an occasional treat, but if you're going to eat chocolate for health, gooey sugar-laden centers shouldn't be part of the program. The high sugar content far outweighs the benefits of the surrounding chocolate. Of course, there's no need to toss out the toffees, creams, and caramels forever. Enjoy your old favorites for special occasions, and eat your new dark chocolate favorites (with dried fruits and nuts, if you like) on the daily plan.

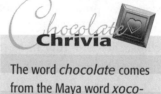

Chocolate Chrivia

The word *chocolate* comes from the Maya word *xocolatl*, pronounced "choco-laahtl." The translation is "bitter water."

Ingredient Dictionary

For the enthusiastic chocolate scientist, I went a step further and researched a large collection of ingredients in chocolate bars of all kinds. The following list comprises the often long and occasionally disgusting (see Shellac) ingredients you may find in your chocolate. The ingredients came right off the labels of actual chocolate bars that I found in both regular and natural grocery stores. "Natural" is a bit misleading, I discovered, which is why it always pays to read the labels.

Reference Key

x   This isn't really ideal but is in quite a few chocolates.

xx   This is what your doctor warned you about.

xxx   You've wandered into the budget chocolate aisle—just say no.

*   Fairly good—most chocolates contain this.

**   Really good—an ingredient in the best chocolates.

***   Amazing—eat this chocolate!

x **Acesulfame K:** A calorie-free synthetic sweetener marketed mostly in Europe under the names Sunett and Sweet One. The *K* stands for potassium, because the sweetener is derived from this mineral. It is 150–200 times sweeter than sugar and does not change its structure in heated conditions, such as in the body (as aspartame does). The majority of studies done on this product show it to be safe, although one can find research to both support and deny this claim. It's not necessary in good-quality chocolate.

x **Artificial flavors:** Who knows what these are? It's a broad category, and using the term is an easy way to avoid listing a long line of ingredients. You'll see it in many chocolates, but it's not your best choice. Stick with natural flavors.

x **Artificial vanilla flavor:** Also called vanillin (with an *n* on the end instead of an *a*). Not the best ingredient but still listed on many chocolate wrappers. The flavor is not nearly as good when compared to natural vanilla. In addition, some people are sensitive to artificial ingredients, which can cause headaches or migraines.

xxx **Aspartame:** There's controversial research all over the board on aspartame, but I believe that it should not be eaten under any conditions. It's toxic to the body, turns to formaldehyde at temperatures higher than 86 degrees Fahrenheit (which will happen in the body, of course), and has been shown to cause numerous adverse symptoms. The approved use of aspartame in the early 1980s came under extremely questionable conditions.

* Beeswax: Whether you're making chocolate, furniture polish, or mustache wax, beeswax appears to have its place. As a food ingredient, it's considered acceptable, although it's not absolutely necessary in chocolate.

x Butter: Being derived from animal products, butter has a bad rap as a food that raises cholesterol. Although this is not the ideal ingredient (cocoa butter is the best fat to look for in chocolate), it's still better than hydrogenated fats.

** Cacao butter: You'd like to see this ingredient in all of the chocolates you eat. Cacao butter (also called cocoa) is a fruit fat and does not raise cholesterol as hydrogenated products do. It's primarily made up of three fats: oleic acid (35%), stearic acid (35%), and palmitic acid (25%). There's also a small amount of linoleic acid (5%).

*** Cacao nibs: Pure cacao beans broken into smaller pieces. After the shells have been winnowed (or blown) away from the beans, they break into these small pieces. You can eat them on cereal, in baked goods, with chocolate, on cottage cheese, or plain. They're very healthy and contain fiber and protein, as well as cocoa butter (about 50%) and cocoa solids.

** Chocolate liquor: Pure cacao beans ground into their finest form. There's no alcohol in chocolate liquor, and you'll often see this ingredient in higher-quality, more expensive bars.

* Citric acid: Like vitamin C, this natural flavoring is often used as a preservative or to bring out the astringent flavor of chocolate.

** Cocoa: Definitely an ingredient you want to see in your chocolate. No cocoa means no chocolate. This is cocoa powder—the result of pressing the cocoa liquor to the extent that it separates the cocoa butter from the cocoa powder.

** **Cocoa beans:** Some labels list "cocoa beans" instead of "cocoa" or "cocoa liquor." Essentially, they mean the same thing, although if you're eating chocolate-covered cocoa beans, you obviously have whole beans.

*** **Cocoa beans, organic:** The same as cocoa beans, but certified organic, meaning that no pesticides or chemicals have been used during any part of the growing or processing.

** **Cocoa butter:** The same thing as cacao butter, listed earlier. Some people differentiate between cacao and cocoa, based on the level of processing. Cacao is unprocessed, whereas cocoa is processed. In that regard, all butter from chocolate would have to be cocoa butter, because the only way to get the butter is to process the cacao beans.

** **Cocoa liquor:** The same as chocolate liquor, described earlier. Various companies list this ingredient in different ways.

*** **Cocoa liquor, organic:** The same as cocoa liquor, but certified organic, meaning that no chemicals or pesticides have been used in any part of the growing or processing.

*** **Cocoa mass:** Another name for chocolate liquor or cocoa liquor.

** **Cocoa processed with alkali:** Also called "dutching," this process mellows the flavor of the beans (which are quite acidic) and darkens the color of the cocoa powder. Most chocolates are made with alkali-processed chocolate, although not all of them mention it on the candy bar wrapper. The alkali process also reduces the antioxidant power of chocolate.

xxx **Corn syrup:** There is a major controversy around the health implications of corn syrup and high fructose corn syrup. Corn syrup is dextrose, a sugar that is three-quarters as sweet as normal sugar. High fructose corn syrup (HFCS) is made from modified corn starch and has a much higher content of fructose sugar. HFCS has been shown to interfere with weight loss by raising triglycerides and shutting down the body's ability to know when it's full, while the less-processed corn syrup apparently does not. It's not a required ingredient for chocolate and certainly not the best sweetener, so look for natural sweeteners such as evaporated cane juice, pure cane sugar, agave, and honey.

xxx **Denatured alcohol:** A flavoring agent. How this ingredient could actually end up in chocolate is incomprehensible. Although the amount contained was probably considered "food grade" and "safe," the actual definition states, "Ethanol that has been rendered toxic or otherwise unfit for consumption." It also doubles as a thinner for shellac. I found this additive contained in a chocolate carried at a popular "natural" grocery store.

* **Dry whole milk:** A flavoring used for milk chocolate. Based on its name, milk chocolate will contain milk products, so you may see this ingredient in your milk chocolates.

** **Evaporated cane juice:** A natural, unprocessed sweetener that is lower on the glycemic index than sugar.

*** **Evaporated cane juice, organic:** The same as evaporated cane juice but certified organic, meaning that no chemicals or pesticides have been used in any part of the growing or processing.

** **Fructose:** A natural fruit sugar, not to be confused with high fructose corn syrup. Fructose is a natural, lower-glycemic sweetener, whereas high fructose corn syrup is not healthy. Get to know the fructose family to save your health—a small variation in wording makes a major difference for your body.

xxx **Glucose syrup:** A cleverly disguised rendition of high fructose corn syrup, this sweetener is derived from cornstarch. A combination of dextrin, maltose, and dextrose, it's best left off this list of ingestible foods.

* **Gum arabic:** The hardened sap of an African tree, often used in cough syrups, jelly beans, cold medicines, and cosmetics. It's very versatile and has many uses. In chocolate, it is most often used for sealing panned confections, such as chocolate-covered nuts.

xxx **High fructose corn syrup:** A man-made, processed syrup made from corn that raises one's blood sugar. It also congests the body's systems by causing the dysfunction of numerous appetite control hormones, including leptin and ghrelin. It's not needed in chocolate or in any diet, for that matter (see also Corn syrup).

xx **Invertase:** An enzyme from saccharaomyces cerevisiale that is used in processing. It's a derivative of saccharide; avoid it.

x **Kolatin gelatin:** A kosher gelling agent; it's not needed in chocolate, although for some reason it was in one particular brand.

* **Lactose:** Sugar that comes from milk. You may see this in milk chocolate, of course. It's natural, but—no surprise here—it's not good for people who are lactose or dairy intolerant.

* **Lactose whey, reduced:** Same as above. Lactose comes from whey, so this is just a fancy way of saying lactose.

xx **Maltitol:** Frequently used in "sugar-free" chocolates, maltitol is responsible for 90 percent of the sweetness of sugar and does contain calories. It has also been shown to raise the blood sugar, although not to the extent of pure sugar. The worst side effect of this sweetener is its tendency to cause indigestion. If you consume too much, just refer to the "Flatulence" section in chapter 6. If you really go overboard, call in sick and cancel all of your meetings. Trust me on this one . . . someone had to do the research.

* **Milk:** Fairly self-explanatory. Of course, you'll see this ingredient or some rendition of it in milk chocolate. As mentioned in other areas of the book, some studies show that the casein in milk binds to the antioxidants in chocolate, rendering them unusable by the body. There's heavy controversy in this area, but it's better to keep your milk and chocolate consumption separate, just to be sure.

* **Milk fat:** Fat from milk. You're not going to get away from milk products when you eat milk chocolate, so if you must have milk chocolate, look for as dark a milk chocolate as possible—

some companies make milk chocolate as high as 40% and even 45% cocoa.

* **Milk powder:** A common ingredient in milk chocolate. Yet it's better to eat a little milk chocolate and stay away from gourmet ice cream, because you'll get considerably less fat in a chocolate bar.

** **Natural bourbon vanilla beans:** Natural vanilla, which is always a good choice. You won't actually find the "beans" in the bar, but rather the vanilla used in the chocolate has come from natural bourbon vanilla beans.

** **Natural flavors:** Who knows what they are, but at least they're natural. Really, though, what is natural? Let's hope you're buying chocolate that gets a little more specific than this.

xxx **Partially hydrogenated palm kernel oil:** See Partially hydrogenated vegetable oil, below.

xxx **Partially hydrogenated sunflower oil:** See Partially hydrogenated vegetable oil, below.

xxx **Partially hydrogenated vegetable oil:** Whenever you see the words *partially hydrogenated* together in the same sentence, steer clear. Hydrogenation adds to the longevity of foods but unfortunately shortens our life spans at the same time. It seems a bit oxymoronic that the product added to foods to make them last longer does double duty by eliminating the very people they're meant to last for. Ultimately, there will be plenty of partially hydrogenated foods on the shelves and no one left to eat them. Whether you see it in chocolate or elsewhere, this ingredient should be avoided like the plague.

x **PGPR, also known as polyglycerol polyricinoleate:** If an ingredient contains more than 46 percent of the alphabet in its name, it's a good idea to stay away from it. Evidently, manufacturers have figured this out and have created less offensive names for these products, such as "PGPR." Actually, "polyglycerol" simply means that it's derived from edible oils (such as sunflower, peanut, corn, etc.), and this particular ingredient is made from castor oil. It helps with viscosity, making chocolate easier to melt in your mouth. It's generally added as a replacement for the far more expensive cocoa butter. If you're not checking the labels yet, you can safely assume you're eating plenty of it because it's in a number of major chocolate brands.

** **Pure cane sugar:** It's hard to say whether this means processed or unprocessed. Unprocessed is ideal, because it is absorbed into the bloodstream more slowly and isn't as bad for your blood sugar as processed white sugar, but this could also be a clever disguise.

* **Salt:** Expands the flavor of chocolate. Sea salt is a recent popular addition to truffles and artisan chocolates, and it has more minerals than the average table salt as well. Salt isn't really needed in chocolate production, but you may see it in these specialty items.

XX **Shellac:** It says "food safe shellac" on the label, but it is a bit of a push to use *shellac*, *food*, and *safe* all in the same sentence. Look for this in many shiny chocolate-covered nuts . . . beauty does have its price. According to *A Consumer's Dictionary for Food Additives* (2004), "lac" is actually the "resinous excretion of certain insects feeding on appropriate host trees." That was only part of the revolting description, which also included adding arsenic to create a glaze that could "safely" be used for candy— up to .4%. Yes, it's legal. Read labels and make smart decisions.

** **Skim milk:** Milk without fat. If you're sensitive to dairy, this is out.

* **Sodium alginate:** A food stabilizer extracted from brown seaweed. This isn't too bad, although it certainly isn't necessary in chocolate.

* **Sodium bicarbonate:** Also known as baking powder or baking soda, this is used in baking as a leavening agent. It's also used to process cocoa, as in alkali-processed chocolate. All things

considered, this doesn't need to be in your chocolate unless you're making brownies or a cake.

x Sorbitan monostearate: An emulsifier sometimes referred to as "synthetic wax." It also has many uses in the plastic, metal, and cosmetics industries and is used in everything from cake mix to hemorrhoid creams . . . it's possibly a little too far outside the chocolate box for health purposes. A popular ingredient in many products but certainly not needed in chocolate.

** Soy lecithin: A natural emulsifier used in a variety of products, from breads, baked goods, and chocolates to hand creams and lotions. You'll see this in most chocolates, because the finicky finished product doesn't like to hold its shape—soy lecithin helps get the job done.

xx Soybean oil, partially hydrogenated: Soybean oil without partial hydrogenation is not too bad on its own. But toss in those two words of destruction, and you're back to fat you don't want to see in your chocolate (see Partially hydrogenated oils).

x Sugar: Processed white sugar is added to most chocolates. It is okay in very low doses, such as in 70% and higher dark chocolate. Ideally, you'd like to see some form of natural sugar in chocolate, as opposed to white sugar, but it's hard to avoid because it's in most chocolates.

* Tapioca dextrin: Tapioca is a thickening agent made from the root of the cassava plant. When combined with dextrin, it can be used as a sealant layer in chocolates. Although the product is natural, good-quality chocolate doesn't require a sealant.

xxx TBHQ, also known as tertiary butylhydroquinone: Another preservative masquerading as a set of initials (see PGPR), a popular new technique that appears to be legal. This preservative is generally added to oils to keep them from oxygenating, and, of course, oils are often added to chocolates. FDA requirements demand that TBHQ content be lower than .02% of the total oil weight because fairly low doses have caused side effects (such as nausea, vomiting, delirium, and even death). Not that you have to worry, however, because manufacturers must comply with the very low percentage regulation. But now you know.

** **Unsweetened chocolate**: This can be a number of things, including processed chocolate with no sugar (such as baking chocolate), cocoa mass, or cocoa liquor.

** **Vanilla**: A natural flavor added to most chocolate. Vanilla enhances the flavor in chocolate, which is why you see it on the ingredient panel so often.

*** **Vanilla pods, Tahitian**: The real thing. If they're from Tahiti, all the better! The vanilla in this chocolate has been extracted from Tahitian vanilla pods. You won't actually find a vanilla pod in the chocolate, but, admittedly, it looks cool on the wrapper.

x **Vanillin**: An artificial vanilla flavor made from eugenol, a synthetic flavoring. It is used in many chocolates and is not good for one's health, although the ingested amount is minute. Some people are very sensitive to artificial flavors, however. As a result, this product is not allowed in nonallergenic products.

x **Vegetable oil**: Olive and canola oils are fine, but when the label simply reads "vegetable oil," it's a safe bet that neither of these two oils is in the chocolate. Look for cocoa butter as the only fat in your chocolate.

* **Whey powder**: Often found in milk chocolate, whey is what's left after the fat and the casein have been extracted from milk—essentially, "powdered milk." It's ideal for chocolate production because liquids that contain water don't mix well with chocolate; the chocolate turns into a giant clump, in what is called "seizing."

* **Whole milk**: Milk that hasn't been defatted. The richest form of milk, generally used in higher-quality milk chocolates. Whole milk contains about 8 grams of fat per serving compared to skim milk (no fat), 1% milk (2.5 grams of fat per serving), and 2% milk (5 grams of fat per serving). This is one reason that

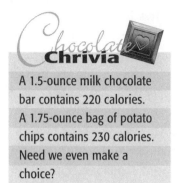

milk chocolate has considerably more fat than dark chocolate does, not to mention a higher percentage of cocoa butter.

Finding Great Chocolate

Now that you have all of this wrapper-reading knowledge, where can you go to use it? Fortunately, it's not as hard to find high-quality chocolate as it was only a few years ago. The good news about "functional chocolate" is that top-quality chocolate sales are increasing, while commercial bars sit idly on shelves awaiting their expiration dates. The trend has not only prompted chocolate stalwarts such as Hershey's, Mars, and Callebaut to step up their higher-percentage collections, but many new chocolatiers are entering the market as well. In fact, there is a larger variety of "healthy" chocolates on the market than ever before, with more brands arriving each year. This makes your search easier.

The most obvious place to look is the candy aisle of the average grocery store, which is home to a selection so vast it could take hours for you to make a decision. This is also where you're most likely to see mass marketers who pay big dollars for shelf space, yet make and sell inferior chocolate products. It's better to look in specialty shops, natural grocers, and fine food stores.

In the United States, large natural-food grocery stores such as Whole Foods Market and Trader Joe's offer diverse and good-quality chocolate selections. The Internet is also an excellent resource. A search for "dark organic chocolate" yields more than 324,000 Web sites worldwide that are devoted to chocolate. One of the best all-inclusive international sites is www.Chocosphere .com. I call it one-stop-choc-shopping: extraordinary international chocolates in a single location. With choices like these at your fingertips, there's no excuse for not finding the perfect high-quality chocolate to suit your every whimsical mood.

Of course, if you live in Europe, you have no idea what I'm talking about because fabulous chocolate is everywhere. Even the smallest grocery stores often devote an entire aisle to chocolate, both right and left sides, all the way down. Thank you, Europe, for setting a standard that all countries should strive for.

The Final Concept

Although it's true that eating chocolate can offer many health benefits, one can nevertheless enjoy too much of a good thing. The final concept is moderation. Many experts advocate eating a little chocolate every day, but this is not carte blanche to eat bonbons for breakfast, truffles for lunch, and chocolate orange wedges for dinner. Moderation is key: one to two ounces a day for good health. More on this later.

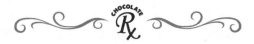

Five

Proper Chocolate Consumption

N ow that you know everything there is to know about fine-quality chocolate, it's time to do your own personal flavor research. You may even have a bar in front of you right now and have already started "investigating." If not, it's time to head to the chocolate stash (you know you have one) and grab some chocolate. At the very least, sneak into the pantry for a handful of chocolate chips. The proper chocolate consumption lesson isn't that difficult and is well worth the effort.

Cultivating Your Chocolate Palate

You've probably never considered whether you eat chocolate properly. I'd been a devout consumer for decades, and the thought never entered my mind. I was amused to discover that there are actually published guidelines to assist with just such a task. Once I read them, I realized I'd been doing it wrong all along. Fortunately, having an imperfect technique didn't appear to affect either my love for chocolate or how much I enjoyed every indulgence. Yet once I began to use the correct procedure, it made all the difference in the world. Even if you have your own technique perfected, take a moment to review this section to make sure you aren't missing anything crucial.

First of all, chocolate tastes best when eaten on an empty stomach. In the event that you ever find you have an empty stomach, this could be the perfect time for a little indulgence. I noticed that the guidelines failed to mention what would happen if you *didn't* have an empty stomach. Conveniently, through personal research I concluded that regardless of the condition of your stomach, chocolate can be eaten without any negative side effects. (Although if you have ulcers, do not eat chocolate on an empty stomach, because it's been reported to occasionally aggravate this condition.)

The next step is for people who are eating more than one kind of chocolate in a single sitting. If you haven't done this yet, I encourage you to splurge—it's time to cross this off the bucket list. You'll need a few different chocolates for this experiment, preferably several brands or those with varying percentages of cocoa. Line them up, from lightest to darkest: white chocolate first (which has no cocoa in it at all), followed by milk chocolate, and finally dark chocolate. Chocolates should be eaten lightest to darkest or based on the amount of cocoa each one contains. Cocoa flavor is quite concentrated, so starting with dark chocolate can overpower your taste buds.

Now you're ready to begin the actual tasting. Pick up the first chocolate and observe it as you would a work of fine art, taking time to examine its beauty and perfection. This step should last anywhere from ten to twenty seconds. The anticipation of your encounter should cause your salivary glands to start

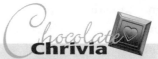

Chrivia

In the United States, Westerners eat more chocolate than do people in the East, and winter is the most popular season to indulge.

working, which will help you taste the chocolate more fully.

Because chocolate melts at 94 degrees Fahrenheit, this step also begins the melting process, which helps release the aromas into the air. Gently wave the chocolate before your nose as you inhale the many tantalizing aromas. Ninety percent of everything you taste comes from your sense of smell, so if you skip this step, you miss a considerable part of the experience.

Slowly place the chocolate on your tongue, allowing your lips to sense the gentle softness of the chocolate's texture. Let it sit in your mouth for a few seconds and begin to melt on your tongue. As you start to chew, swirl the chocolate around our entire mouth.

The idea is to allow all of your mouth to experience the chocolate. Some research claims that the tongue has four zones of taste buds—salt, sour, bitter, and sweet—so the chocolate will stimulate unique flavor sensations in each zone. Yet more recent research suggests that the entire tongue tastes most flavors and that there are taste buds on the soft palate and the upper epiglottis as well. Why take chances, though? Swirl the chocolate around for your own benefit, zone or no zones. Chocolate has more than four hundred flavor compounds, and once you slow down and focus, you'll start to notice more of them.

Continue chewing as you swirl, but don't swallow just yet. Take a moment to press the chocolate onto the roof of your mouth with your tongue, savoring one last moment of melting and flavorful euphoria. Relax, breathe deeply, and take in the lingering cacophony of sensations. Once you've completed this final step of delicious enjoyment, swallow at last. Note the flavors as they fade away—you may find something different that you didn't taste while it was in your mouth.

Before indulging in your next chocolate, rinse your mouth thoroughly with water, light tea, or wine to prepare the palate for the next unique experience. Some connoisseurs insist on rinsing only with water, because wine or tea can desensitize the taste buds. Yet others recommend consuming chocolate with wine, which, when paired properly, can offer a unique culinary experience. It's up to you to choose whose side you're on—fortunately, everyone wins because chocolate is involved in both cases. Read chapter 8, "Chocolate and Wine Pairing," before you make a firm decision.

When you're ready, move to the next confection for another go-round, and repeat the process exactly as previously described. You may stop when you've reached the necessary level of satiation or when all of the chocolate is gone, whichever comes first.

Once you've acquired the skills of an advanced connoisseur, you'll be able to discern a wide variety of bean flavors without even referring to the wrapper. Chocolate picks up the nuances of the land where it's grown. Remember, there are more than four hundred different flavor compounds in chocolate. Be prepared for an entertaining variety of flavor sensations, such as spices, peppers, mango, pineapple, raspberry, cream, espresso, blueberry, lavender, almond, coffee, and even tobacco. See the Chocolate Flavor Wheel in chapter 8 for dozens of possibilities.

After you've fine-tuned your tasting skills, the extreme chocolate enthusiast's next step is learning how to identify beans by country, based on their flavors. "Single origin" chocolates are those made with beans exclusively from one country or region.

Most chocolates are blends, but the popularity of "single origin" is on the rise, as people expand their chocolate knowledge.

Bean Flavor Profiles

The flavors listed here are general for each country and will not be found in every "single origin" chocolate. The flavors vary from region to region within the country, so various brands have unique flavors, depending on where the beans came from. The following list will help you get started.

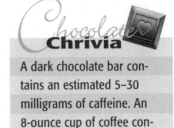

Chocolate Chrivia

A dark chocolate bar contains an estimated 5–30 milligrams of caffeine. An 8-ounce cup of coffee contains 100–150 milligrams.

Africa

Ghana: Similar to Ivory Coast, with classic cocoa flavors, bold, forward, floral in some areas

Ivory Coast: Rich, intense cocoa, tobacco, leather

Madagascar: Light citrus, tangerine, bright acidity, exotic fruit, wine, raspberry, raisin, hazelnut, berry, clove, cedar

São Tomé: Robust, fruity, forward, bold, deep chocolate, roasted coffee, cinnamon, vanilla

Tanzania: Creamy, fruity, floral

Asia

Bali: Honey, figs, spicy, licorice, nut, gentle flavor

Java: Acidic, leather, smoky, balanced cocoa flavors

Caribbean

Dominican Republic: Earthy, tobacco, spice, fruity, orange, grapefruit, bergamot

Grenada: Light, acidic, citrus fruits, orange, lemon, dry wood

Haiti: Strong acidity, spicy, cocoa

Jamaica: Peaches, pineapple, cedar, rum

Trinidad: Well-balanced, spicy, cinnamon

Mexico, Central America

Costa Rica: Fruity, balanced cocoa, uniquely floral

Mexico: Bright acidity, lemon

Panama: Roasted cocoa, fruit

South America

Bolivia: Light and fresh, lemon, grapefruit, vanilla, plum

Brazil: Balanced cocoa, vanilla, bold, subtle fruit

Colombia: Coffee, nutty, fruity, floral, mild acidity

Ecuador: Coffee, licorice, spice, vanilla, herbal, jasmine

Venezuela: Complex flavors, nutty, sweet, red fruit, apricot, ripe plum, cherry

Keep in mind that even if you've been eating chocolate incorrectly for years, no harm will come of it. My own technique involved moving directly from sliding the chocolate into my mouth (although not slowly, as advised) to cleansing my palate in preparation for the next confection. The discovery of fifteen missing steps was a shocking surprise. Of course, it's never too late to change. Once you've started to make step-by-step adjustments, you may realize that some of those steps are rather valuable. Pass the wine, please.

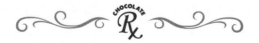

Six

Chocolate Remedies

OR YEARS, I ATTEMPTED to control my chocolate habit through abstinence, an effort that proved to be extremely agonizing at times. So, I was delighted when I discovered that chocolate has the power to heal. It didn't take me long to make sure I properly addressed every conceivable health problem.

The premise is very simple—find your ailment and follow the chocolate recommendation. It's best to use a little common sense while self-medicating. If you suffer from a host of problems, it won't do much good to try to resolve everything at once.

Although having a little chocolate is healthy, eating ten of the recommended bars in a single day is likely to induce an entirely new set of disorders you may not be prepared to deal with.

As mentioned in chapter 5, I suggest eating one to two ounces of dark chocolate per day for health. I gave a presentation about the health benefits of chocolate at a cardiologist's office who was advising his patients about healthy chocolate consumption—he also suggested one ounce per day. Finding your ideal dose might require you to do a little more research. After all, who better than you to determine how much chocolate you can eat per day?

One more clarification before moving on: what exactly is an ounce? How many times have you been instructed to eat an ounce of something, and you have no idea how much that is? Most of us have a general idea of what twelve ounces of beer looks like, but what about an ounce of chocolate? What if you accidentally eat a quarter pound of chocolate under the mistaken belief that you're only indulging in a mere ounce? Use the following simple guidelines to avoid possible overindulgence:

28 grams = 1 ounce

100 grams = 3.5 ounces

1 ounce = a little more than half of a regular grocery store candy bar.

1½ ounces = the size of most regular grocery store bars.

2 ounces = the size of most good-quality chocolate bars.

4 ounces = more chocolate than you should be eating per day, also known as a quarter pound of chocolate.

When in doubt, read the wrapper. The size is always listed on the bar.

The ailments are alphabetized and divided into two parts: "Recommendation" and "Supporting Evidence." The

"Recommendation" section consists of chocolate bars with an assortment of different ingredients, all carefully chosen to help alleviate the listed ailment. The Supporting Evidence section presents results gathered from current research showing how chocolate can help with the ailment at hand. Most of the recommendations call for dark chocolate, but I've included a few milk chocolate selections for the sake of variety. Keep in mind that dark chocolate is the best choice when you're eating chocolate for its health benefits.

You may become completely healthy and have no further need to consult this book. If so, consider following a preventative program of eating a small amount of healthy chocolates every day. (Unfortunately, insurance companies do not currently cover this new preventative health-care plan.) And don't let your inquiry stop with this book. Keep up with experts who are continually researching the many benefits of chocolate. With thousands of ongoing studies under way, undoubtedly the best news is yet to come.

The recommended chocolates are simply suggestions. Feel free to exchange the recommendation for your own chocolate remedy wherever you like, provided that it meets the ingredient guidelines in chapter 4. Of course, you can venture outside the guidelines. Just keep in mind the "healthy chocolate for health benefits" concept.

Over time, I predict that what happened to me will happen to you: your extraordinary new outlook on chocolate will prove monumentally beneficial. People will wonder why you're looking so radiant and will demand to know what you're doing. You may even become the life of the party. And with your new and astonishing knowledge about the benefits of one of the world's most loved foods, you'll save countless others from a lifetime of deprivation.

And now the remedies.

ADD / ADHD

Recommendation

Take 1 ounce 75% dark chocolate almond bark (ideally sweetened with evaporated cane juice or agave nectar) midmorning when attention is likely to start waning. Avoid caffeine, vending machines, and the office doughnut box.

Supporting Evidence

The relationship of diet to attention deficit disorder (ADD) and attention deficit hyperactivity disorder (ADHD) has been confirmed for quite some time, although it is still considered controversial. How someone could presume that food intake does *not* affect concentration is slightly beyond belief, but, fortunately, health-care practitioners are finally starting to embrace the diet-attention concept.

Generally, people who suffer from ADD and ADHD are instructed to stay away from sugar, at the very least, so it's important to eat dark chocolate—a minimum of 75% cocoa to ensure more nutrient value and less sugar content. Chocolate's main benefit to the brain comes from its high magnesium content, which is also the brain's most prevalent mineral. Magnesium is essential for the brain to convert glucose into energy, for helping to clear away metabolic wastes, and to use essential fats to construct the brain's cell membranes. The number of ways that magnesium benefits the brain fills an entire book. Consider reading *The Miracle of Magnesium* by Dr. Carolyn Dean for additional information.

People who have severe magnesium deficiencies often suffer from attention disorders, apathy, irritability, depression, and confusion. Chocolate is one of the highest natural sources of magnesium of all foods on the planet. Almonds are rich in magnesium as well. The two together can supply as much as

30 percent of your daily magnesium requirement. If you're really suffering, consider adding other magnesium-rich foods to your diet, such as sunflower seeds, cashews, broccoli, and spinach.

Whether or not you suffer from ADD or ADHD, it's still quite likely that you're magnesium-deficient. According to www .NaturalNews.com, a government study published in 2008 reported that 68 percent of Americans don't consume enough magnesium, and 19 percent don't even consume half of the daily requirement. Magnesium is required in more than three hundred enzymatic reactions in the body, so you might consider adding extra magnesium to your diet in addition to a few squares of chocolate.

Allergies

Recommendation

Take 2 squares dark or milk chocolate, every 6 hours as needed, while drinking ginger tea. Do not exceed 12 squares in any 24-hour period. Children under 12 should take half of the dose.

Supporting Evidence

Chocolate contains theobromine, which has recently been shown to offer the same cough-suppressing advantages as codeine (see "Cough," later in the chapter). Although the theobromine content in chocolate is relatively small, its effects have still been measured in the blood subsequent to people ingesting even small amounts of chocolate. In fact, nearly every element in chocolate that benefits your health is present in relatively small doses, but it's the combination of all of the elements in a single food source that helps the body.

The recommended ginger tea offers significant relief as well. Ginger contains anti-inflammatory properties. It's long been used by traditional healers to help control a variety of health problems, including allergies and other respiratory conditions. It's a natural antihistamine, as well as a decongestant, and it dilates constricted bronchial tubes, thus offering relief to the sufferer. A number of chocolate companies already offer ginger in their selections, making your quest for relief very convenient.

Are you allergic to chocolate? In a study of eighty-one people who believed they were allergic to chocolate, researchers found only one person with an actual chocolate allergy. Another study of five hundred people who stated they were allergic to chocolate revealed that only one person had a true allergic reaction. According to a prominent allergist at the National Jewish Medical Research Center in Denver, thirty years of allergy testing for chocolate revealed fewer than thirty-five cases of actual chocolate allergies. This is not to say that chocolate allergies don't exist, but they aren't nearly as prevalent as one might think.

It's possible that some people try to convince themselves that they're allergic to chocolate merely as an excuse to stay away from it—this is certainly a form of self-torture we should all avoid. Of course, if you're positively allergic to chocolate, you may want to pass this book on to a friend.

Occasionally, people deprive themselves of chocolate because they're allergic to dairy. Yet because there's no dairy in chocolate to begin with, the only way to get it is to add it in. If you read the ingredient label, it's easy to find good-quality dark chocolate that doesn't contain dairy products. Of course, you will see dairy in milk chocolate, but, ideally, dark chocolate should be free of milk products. If your chocolate is suspect, this is the perfect time to review the section in chapter 4 called "Wrapper Reading 101." Once you know the ground rules, you can make choices to support your health.

Alzheimer's Disease

Recommendation

Take 1 ounce 70%+ dark chocolate with acai and blueberry once daily for the rest of your life. Optional: enjoy it with ½ cup acai juice with a dash of lemon juice or the juice from ¼ freshly squeezed lemon.

Supporting Evidence

According to a 2009 report published by the Alzheimer's Association (www.alz.org), every seventy seconds someone is diagnosed with Alzheimer's disease. An estimated twelve million people suffer from Alzheimer's disease worldwide, a number that is projected to go up as the human life span increases. Because the rate of Alzheimer's doubles for every five years of age, people who live past the age of ninety have a 50 percent chance of developing the disease. Unfortunately, there's no way to tell which side of the coin you'll fall on, but you can swing the odds in your favor by paying attention to what you eat now.

One cause of Alzheimer's is a build-up of excess amyloid plaques, proteins that coagulate in the brain, cause blockages, and reduce normal brain functioning. Researchers at Cornell University discovered that a diet rich in antioxidant foods helps protect the brain against amyloid plaque damage. Of particular interest, one of the antioxidants in chocolate called epicatechin was able to cross the blood-brain barrier and help protect the brain. A study from the Vanderbilt School of Medicine confirms the importance of antioxidant consumption. The nine-year study of 1,836 people showed that those who consumed fruit and vegetable juices at least three times a week had a 75 percent lower risk of developing Alzheimer's than did those who drank them only one to two times per week.

Acai and blueberries are recommended because both are extremely high in antioxidants, not to mention that they taste delicious with chocolate. Acai is a powerfully potent, antioxidant-rich fruit that hails from South America. It has long been a staple in the Amazon region and has just recently begun to cross the borders into mainstream use all over the world. Acai juice, on its own, tastes a little like cough syrup (my opinion, of course), but blend it into a top-quality dark chocolate, and it's like a good cabernet sauvignon paired with dark mint chocolate—unexpected perfection.

Blueberries are included with the recommendation, because they've also been shown to boost brain function in numerous studies. In a study from *Nutrition & Neuroscience*, researchers showed that people who were given blueberries daily for four weeks had improved decision making, reported less pain, had higher energy levels, experienced better sleep, and had more mental acuity. The control group (which was not given blueberries) showed no changes.

One other tip to help preserve your brain—cut back on canned soda and canned beverages. Many of these drinks contain excessive levels of aluminum, another toxin found at high levels in the brains of Alzheimer's patients. It's best to enjoy your chocolate with a glass of red wine or a cup of green tea. Really now, it won't be that difficult . . . give it a try.

Andropause (Male Menopause)

Recommendation

Take ¼ cup dark chocolate chips and a handful of peanuts with a mug of light lager, preferably while relaxing in front of a ball game or hanging out with the guys on the back porch. Sample personal favorite beers and various chocolate chip brands for maximum effectiveness. Do not indulge in an excessive number of pairings on a single day, or side effects will take hold, such as a snappish significant other, weight gain, and a possible hangover.

Supporting Evidence

As much as men would like to deny the existence of male menopause, statistics speak louder than opinions. In fact, to this day, the term *andropause* is not recognized by the World Health Organization as a medical classification, leading one to conclude that men over forty must be in charge there. Nonetheless, a quick review of post-forty male physiological functioning will help convince the skeptic.

In the ultimate bait-and-switch, the same male hormone that caused all kinds of issues as it surged in youth is now creating other problems as its level subsides. The culprit is testosterone, generating a classic case of "can't live with it, can't live without it." Andropause brings many of the same symptoms that women experience in menopause—loss of libido, impaired memory, hot flashes, inability to concentrate, mood swings, night sweats, depression, and, of course, the most dramatic symptom for men: erectile dysfunction.

Women have dealt with hormone fluctuations for twenty-five years or more by this point, but many men are caught off-guard by the sudden change. Erratic reactions are the norm, including the apparent belief that dashing off to buy a Porsche will somehow curtail the effects. In the event that you're not able to afford this strategy (which is still under debate among women as to its value), a more effective plan includes eating nutrient-dense foods that help restore hormone imbalance.

According to an article in *Men's Health*, men lose approximately 1 percent of their testosterone per year beginning around age forty, although it starts as soon as the early thirties for some men. The article lists a number of ways to raise testosterone naturally, such as weight loss (excess weight carries estrogen, the "female" hormone); avoiding super-high-protein diets, which can decrease natural testosterone levels; keeping alcohol consumption to three drinks a day or less (alcohol compromises the testes' production of male hormones); and getting a good night's sleep, among other suggestions.

The article also recommended eating nuts, which is why the recommendation includes eating a handful of nuts each day. Monounsaturated fats are essential for hormone production. They are present in many nuts, as well as in certain oils, such as olive oil and canola oil. Peanuts are part of the recommendation because they are one of the nuts that is highest in monounsaturated fats and are good for this remedy.

Anemia

Recommendation

Take 4 squares dark chocolate with almonds on an empty stomach or any other time you feel like taking it, up to a maximum of 12 squares in a given day. Optional: 10 additional almonds (without chocolate), taken at any time. Chew thoroughly before swallowing.

Supporting Evidence

Anemia is a condition in which the amount of red blood cells in the bloodstream falls to a very low level. Without enough red cells, the body is unable to carry the oxygen that is needed to maintain healthy tissues and organs. Iron helps build red blood cells, and a deficiency in this mineral can lead to anemia. Eating foods that are rich in iron can help reduce the possibility of your becoming anemic.

A good-quality bar of dark chocolate provides approximately 7.5 percent of your daily iron requirement. Adding 3.5 ounces of almonds brings the total up to 29 percent, and almonds perform double duty. Not only do they boost the daily iron percentage, but they also contain copper (approximately 1.15 milligrams per 100 grams of chocolate). When combined with the vitamins and the iron in chocolate, copper acts as a catalyst for the formation of new blood cells. If you're really feeling industrious, melt the chocolate and the almonds together (on very low heat) in an iron pot. A report published in *Food Chemistry* confirmed that cooking foods in iron pots can raise the iron content significantly.

The recommendation to "chew thoroughly" is just as important as enjoying a little chocolate. Nuts are very fibrous and a challenge for the body to digest. How often do you grab a handful of nuts, chew for a few seconds, and then reach for the second handful, while forcing the barely chewed glob down your throat with some kind of drink? Half-chewed nuts are difficult for the stomach to digest, but a well-chewed nut arrives in the stomach ready for absorption. People with anemia often have problems absorbing the nutrients in food, and proper chewing can be an excellent place to start to deal with this.

This is where you can step in with a little personal research. The next time you reach for the chocolate and the nuts, pay attention to how you eat them. And remember: if at first you don't succeed, chew, chew again.

Antioxidant Assistance

Recommendation

Take 4 squares intense dark organic chocolate (65%+) or 6–10 chocolate-covered goji berries throughout the day; repeat daily as you wish, up to a maximum of 1.75 ounces of chocolate in a 24-hour period. Optional: try dark chocolate with dried apricots.

Supporting Evidence

When it comes to chocolate, "high in antioxidants" is probably the most often heard praise. Chapter 3 goes into more detail, but a quick review will remind you why the word *chocolate* has become synonymous with *antioxidants*.

According to the Whole Food Supplement Guide (www .whole-foods-supplement-guide.com), the best sources of antioxidants come from fresh fruits and vegetables. Chocolate generally tops the antioxidant charts because it's not only a fruit, but, rather, it's made from the *ground seeds of a fruit tree*—the most nutrient-dense element of the fruit.

Red wine is also very rich in antioxidants. As such, many doctors advise drinking a 4-ounce glass a day for health. Yet chocolate contains twice the antioxidants of wine by weight because all of the liquid and the fats have been extracted from the cocoa beans. With red wine, the amount of antioxidants is diluted by the liquid in the wine. But chocolate starts with cocoa powder. Pure cocoa powder is twice as antioxidant dense as 70% dark chocolate, so add a little to your baked goods whenever you cook.

A report published in the *Journal of Agricultural and Food Chemistry* states that "chocolate is the third highest daily per capita antioxidant source" in the U.S. diet. This statistic borderline qualifies chocolate as its own food group, but to benefit, you must eat dark chocolate. Remember that *all* of chocolate's benefits are in the cocoa powder. There's nothing at all in the cocoa butter—sorry, white chocolate lovers.

Apricots are recommended because they're rich in vitamin A, which is considered to be one of the most powerful of all of the vitamins for immune system assistance. In his book *Encyclopedia of Nutritional Supplements*, author Michael T. Murray cites research comparing the life spans of various species with respect to concentrations of carotenoids (vitamin A) in the blood. The research shows that as the concentration of vitamin A increases, the maximum potential life span increases as well. Of course, carrots are also an extraordinary source of vitamin A, but personal research indicates that they don't pair as well with chocolate as apricots do. Still, feel free to experiment.

Antiwrinkle Assistance

Recommendation

Take 6 squares dark organic chocolate, one at a time, with a glass of red wine. Enjoy them at home while hosting a spa party with the girls, the guys, or both. Apply a dark chocolate mask (instructions on how to make the mask follow). An entertaining chocolate-themed movie is optional. Repeat this treatment monthly.

Supporting Evidence

The recent explosion of chocolate-based skin-care products confirms that chocolate is no longer limited to consumption. It's now acceptable for the face and the body as well. I refer to this as the calorie-free chocolate solution for skeptics who will never adopt a daily chocolate regimen—this one is guaranteed not to pack on the pounds. You simply put it on your skin, instead of in your mouth, and the results speak for themselves. If after some time you find the mere smell of chocolate on your skin too torturous, however, reconsider the inside-out program: a little on the face, a little in the mouth.

Perhaps you're questioning the logic of applying chocolate to the face, because it's rumored to cause acne. Yet just like everything else in life, correct application is the key. Here are just few of the facts quoted from Ecco Bella, a company that makes a very nice chocolate mask: "This chocolate mask treatment is naturally pure and rich in iron, magnesium, vitamins and antioxidants. . . . These nutrients nourish and cleanse your skin while leaving it softer and smoother than ever." When you participate with a group of friends, you'll get the fabulous benefit of laughing hysterically when you see how lovely everyone looks in his or her fresh and skin-friendly dark chocolate mask.

Next, apply a little pure cocoa butter to problem areas. Just like the mask, this product is loaded with vitamins, minerals, and more wrinkle-fighting antioxidants. A report published in the *International Journal of Cosmetic Science* demonstrated improved skin tone and elasticity from cocoa butter application.

Cocoa butter is available in most variety and grocery stores, but the cocoa mask can be a little more difficult to come by. If you can't find one, simply make your own chocolate mask by adding chocolate to your favorite skin-care product. Necessary skills include microwave operation and stirring with a spoon in a bowl. Studies (mine in particular) have confirmed that children as young as seven and nine are capable of such a project.

To do this at home: melt baking chocolate in the microwave (thirty seconds at a time on low heat in a microwaveable glass bowl). Stop heating the chocolate when there are a few solid pieces left, and stir to finish the job. This will keep the chocolate from becoming too hot. One you have a semicool bowl of melted chocolate, add a little of it to your favorite face cream in a separate bowl. No recipe is required—this is trial and error: a little of this, a little of that. The key is to get the mixture to a consistency that will not drip off your face.

Another option is to use pure cocoa powder in your own skin-care cream. Make sure to use pure baking cocoa powder and *not* hot chocolate mix, which contains sugar and preservatives.

You might also invest in a copy of *Chocolate Bliss* by Susie Norris, a do-it-yourself-chocolate-spa book with enticing recipes such as cocoa body lotion, melt-away chocolate massage oil, and even chocolate soap. If you'd rather have someone else do the prep work, visit Sweet Beauty, a Web site devoted to organic chocolate spa treatments (www.sweetbeautyspa.com).

For those who opt to eat a little chocolate, as well as use it on the skin, keep in mind that the darker your selection, the more health benefits you'll receive. Dark chocolate contains considerably less sugar than milk chocolate, another major benefit to the skin. Sugar binds to collagen, making it stiff and inflexible. Over time, this adds wrinkles to your face and other sensitive skin areas. A study from the *Journal of Nutrition* reported encouraging results for the skin as well. Women who drank 100 milligrams of a chocolate flavanol-rich beverage daily for twelve weeks had higher skin tolerance to ultraviolet light exposure. Their skin was also thicker and denser and had more hydration and less scaling.

Take the leap, and buy only the best chocolate for the antiwrinkle program. When you spend a little extra on what goes in your mouth and on your skin, you'll end up spending much less than you would on antiwrinkle treatments. You can eat a lot of great-quality chocolate for the cost of laser skin rejuvenation. Now, off you go to the spa.

Anxiety

Recommendation

Take 1 ounce dark chocolate with vanilla and dried blueberries and a cup of herbal berry tea, preferably just before dinner and not too close to bedtime. Repeat daily for 56 days.

Supporting Evidence

Anxiety is an inability to cope with the stresses of life as they unfold, and unfold they do! Interestingly, a report from the Johns Hopkins Medical Institution demonstrated that people who are prone to anxiety are more sensitive to bodily changes than those who aren't. Two people can experience exactly the same event, and one handles it easily and effectively, while the other has a complete a breakdown or a full panic attack. What is the difference?

One reason some people aren't equipped to handle the challenges of life is that their adrenals are overstressed, a symptom caused by an improperly functioning pituitary gland. The pituitary needs an adequate supply of magnesium to function properly, and chocolate is one of the richest sources of natural magnesium of all natural foods. Magnesium also helps the muscles relax, offering a double dose of positive effects for people who are prone to excessive anxiety.

How many times have you heard, "It's not that bad, it's just your interpretation of events that makes you anxious"? You want to smack the person who says it. But why not simply indulge in a little chocolate instead? It's much less of a hassle in the long run, and it won't come back to sue you later, which could effectively cause more anxiety.

Fifty-six days of following the recommendation are suggested because, according to researchers at the University of Grenada in Spain, this is how many days of chocolate consumption it took to bring magnesium levels back to normal in magnesium-deficient rats. If you find that you have favorable results, consider extending your study beyond 56 days, perhaps for a lifetime. Another option would be to add 250 milligrams of magnesium per day for 56 days. This strategy accomplishes the same effect faster than chocolate does, but why not do both, for your anxiety-reducing pleasure?

Arthritis

Recommendation

Take 4 squares dark chocolate with dried tart cherries (and optional hazelnuts) every 4 hours, as needed, to reduce pain and increase chocolate euphoria. Take with or without meals. Do not exceed a maximum of 12 squares in any 24-hour period (or 2 ounces, for those whose "square" is on the larger side). Attend water aerobics once a week.

Supporting Evidence

According to a report from the Centers for Disease Control (CDC), approximately 33 percent of the U.S. population now suffers from arthritis, up 60 percent during the last twelve years. It's considered one of the most common health problems in the United States, affecting as many as seventy million adults. Incidence is higher among women than men, is higher among whites than blacks, and is more common for overweight, physically inactive adults (www.AllAboutArthritis.com).

A report published in the *Journal of Pharmacology and Experimental Therapeutics* showed that polyphenols significantly reduce the possibility of developing some forms of arthritis. Polyphenols are plant chemicals, powerful antioxidants that work tirelessly to rid the body of destructive free radicals, which are a primary cause of arthritis. Polyphenols are very plentiful in chocolate.

Cherries are included in the recommendation because they contain a specific antioxidant called anthocyanin, known for its ability to block inflammatory compounds called prostaglandins. The research, reported in the *Journal of Natural Products*, specifically referenced "tart" cherries, as opposed to sweet cherries. So adding maraschino cherries to your hot fudge sundae will not count, for either the cherries or the chocolate. If you follow the recommendation, however, you'll be in good hands because anthocyanin is also contained in chocolate, so adding *tart cherries* to your *dark chocolate* doubles the weapons in your war on arthritis.

Eating chocolate with nuts is recommended because nuts assist with calcium absorption and help prevent the body from becoming calcium-deficient. A number of studies have shown that a deficiency in calcium can contribute to arthritis.

Kick the recommendation into full gear with a water aerobics class. According to physical therapist Doreen Stiskall, if you're standing in a pool of water up to your shoulders, only 10 percent of your body weight is affecting your joints. This not only makes exercising much less painful to arthritis sufferers, but the water also offers resistance to help build strength. Stiskall, who recently helped the Arthritis Foundation overhaul its water aerobics program, recommends finding a facility with warm water (a minimum of 83 degrees F), a knowledgeable instructor, a program that gradually builds skills and increases the level of activity, and a good social atmosphere.

Note: to increase the likelihood of finding a positive social atmosphere, bring the chocolate with tart dried cherries to class.

Asthma

Recommendation

Take ½ dark chocolate bar with mint and 1 cup peppermint tea. Read a good book, and repeat as necessary until you feel better. Do not exceed a maximum of 1 bar per day.

Supporting Evidence

Asthma is a respiratory disorder generally believed to be caused by an allergic reaction that involves immune system dysfunction. When the body senses that it is under attack, it releases hista-mines to combat foreign substances such as dust, pollen, and some types of food. In an overresponsive body, histamines send an excessive rush of blood and lymph fluid to the affected area, causing an inflammation of the lungs and impeding breathing.

Chocolate contains a natural plant chemical called proantho-cyanidin, which is both an antioxidant and an anti-inflammatory. Proanthocyanidin is used in vitamins and medicines that are specially formulated to alleviate arthritis, another inflammatory disease. Proanthocyanidin can actually help block the body's release of histamines, thus lessening the side effects of an asthmatic allergic reaction (www.AsthmaWorld.org).

The small amount of caffeine in certain chocolates may be beneficial as well. Caffeinated foods and beverages can help dilate bronchial tubes and make breathing easier. Those who suffer from asthma should also make a note to commit to eating dark chocolate, rather than milk chocolate. More than one study has confirmed that the milk protein "casein" is an allergen that can trigger both asthma and sinus problems. Two excellent resources for more information on this particular subject are top-selling weight-loss and nutrition books *8 Minutes in the Morning* by Jorge Cruise and *Eating Well for Optimum Health* by nutrition and health expert Dr. Andrew Weil.

Peppermint tea is suggested as part of the plan because it helps clear the breathing passages. Peppermint oil has been used for centuries as a decongestant because it relaxes nasal passages and even reduces pain. It's often found in cough syrups, ointments, nasal decongestants, and inhalants. But why go to all of that medicinal trouble? You can enjoy many of the same benefits by simply eating a mint chocolate bar and drinking a cup of mint tea.

Blood Sugar Control: Hypoglycemia

Recommendation

Take 4 squares 70%+ dark chocolate and cinnamon, with or without almonds, hazelnuts, or pecans, along with 8 ounces

water or skim milk. Consume these after the lunch meal.
Optional: may also be taken as a midmorning snack.

Supporting Evidence

Dark chocolate is an excellent choice when you are considering
snacks that will keep your blood sugar under control. It contains fat, fiber, protein, and a relatively low level of sugar, so it's
absorbed into the bloodstream quite slowly. Follow these guidelines to ensure maximum success.

Although it's true that chocolate supposedly tastes better on
an empty stomach (see chapter 5), this is not the ideal way to
eat chocolate when you're attempting to keep your blood sugar
stable. Instead, you should eat it after a meal, preferably one in
which you've consumed a healthy portion of protein (20 grams
or more). Protein acts as a stabilizer for blood sugar because it's
absorbed into the bloodstream very slowly. It balances foods that
cause blood sugar to rise, such as sugars and processed carbohydrates. And even though a 50-gram dark chocolate bar contains
3 grams of protein, you're still better off eating chocolate after a
protein-rich meal.

Chocolate also contains chromium, a mineral associated with
controlling blood sugar. A comprehensive report in *Diabetes
Care* evaluated more than eighty different studies on blood
sugar and chromium and concluded that adding chromium
to the daily diet has a positive effect on glucose metabolism.
It may even help increase your ability to properly metabolize
cholesterol.

Adding nuts will also help keep your blood sugar levels low.
Nuts contain fat, and, like protein, fat reduces the rate at which
sugar is absorbed into the bloodstream. If you were given a choice
between eating a bowl of processed or refined cereal (almost any
brand) or a dark chocolate bar, the dark chocolate bar would
raise your blood sugar less. In fact, nearly every processed cereal

raises the blood sugar substantially, while a dark chocolate bar with nuts comes in quite low, at 34 on the glycemic index (GI) scale. (See appendix B for a brief description of the glycemic index, how it works, and how to use it to lose weight.)

Cinnamon is another part of the recommendation because recent research shows that it helps metabolize glucose. In one study, participants with type 2 diabetes were given a quarter teaspoon of cinnamon twice daily. They experienced a reduction in both blood sugar level and bad cholesterol. Another study reported by the American Diabetic Association showed similar results. Subjects who were given 1, 3, and 6 grams of cinnamon all had reduced serum glucose, triglycerides, and LDL cholesterol.

Both chocolate and cinnamon contain proanthocyanidin, an antioxidant that appears to activate the insulin receptors in cells. At the L'Aquila University in Italy, participants were given 100 grams of dark chocolate every day for fifteen days. At the end of the study, the subjects had lower blood pressure and were more receptive to insulin.

Caffeine Withdrawal

Recommendation

Take 1 ounce 65% dark chocolate or 5–10 chocolate-covered coffee beans any time of day with a cup of coffee or a caffeinated beverage of your choice. Limit to one chocolate serving per day. The total quantity of chocolate-covered beans may vary, according to the task at hand.

Supporting Evidence

Chocolate has long been credited as a pick-me-up food because it contains caffeine, but the amount of caffeine in chocolate is virtually insignificant. A 2-ounce chocolate bar might contain up to 20 milligrams of caffeine, but it's closer to 0–5 milligrams. Most chocolate contains hardly any caffeine, although content varies significantly depending on where it's grown. For example, beans from the Forastero tree, which account for as much as 70 percent of the world's chocolate, contain virtually no caffeine at all.

But don't lose faith in using chocolate in your pick-me-up plan just yet. The confusion arises because people assume that the lift they experience comes from caffeine. Yet it's actually from a similar stimulant called theobromine, which is closely config- ured to caffeine but milder and a little less agitating.

Still, quite a number of people have told me they can't eat chocolate in the evening because it keeps them awake. Unless it's a dessert emergency, I rarely eat it after 4 P.M. for the same reason. If you find yourself wide awake all night after a chocolate indulgence, you might want to follow the pre-4 P.M. chocolate plan. If it's too late and you're up at 2 A.M., consider visiting www.ChatChewandChocolate.com to connect with your herd.

A caffeinated drink is part of the recommendation because if you really have a thing for caffeine, you'd be hard-pressed to eat enough chocolate to get a caffeine buzz. If you did eat that much, you'd likely find yourself referring to the weight- loss section of this book. For die-hard caffeine addicts, it's better to include a caffeinated beverage as recommended. A few companies offer chocolate selections with the espresso flavor already added in, to assure adequate energy for your next endeavor, whether it's shopping, driving cross coun- try, or cycling twenty miles on your lunch hour. Extremists (you know who you are) would do well to visit www .TheChocolateTherapist.com for a bag of 72% dark chocolate– covered espresso beans.

Cancer

Recommendation

Take ½ dark chocolate bar with or without almonds daily for the rest of your life. Optional: 1 ounce dark chocolate–covered orange peel.

Supporting Evidence

Cancer is caused by cells multiplying uncontrollably, destroying healthy tissues, and taking over the body. Consult any book on which foods are best to eat to help combat the effects of cancer, and all of the advice is in sync—eat whole, unprocessed foods, preferably fresh fruits and vegetables.

Plants contain chemical compounds called polyphenols, many of which are highly protective antioxidants that provide a powerful boost to the immune system and help fight disease. There are two types of polyphenols associated with chocolate and cocoa. The first one is flavonoids, which are divided into flavanols (specifically, flavan-3-ols) and proanthocyanidins (which are linked flavanol units). It also contains flavonols, which include catechin, epicatechin, and quercetin. A number of reports show that these compounds are particularly powerful allies in the fight against cancer.

An Italian study on cancer cell behavior demonstrated that certain polyphenols help regulate "apoptosis," a programmed cell death that ceases to function properly in cancerous cells. At the University of Hawaii's Cancer Research Center, volunteers whose diets contained the highest amounts of flavonoids showed a 40 to 50 percent reduction in lung cancer. In a Finnish study, a twenty-four-year investigation of ten thousand people confirmed that people who regularly ate the largest quantities of flavonoids showed a 20 percent reduction in developing all types of cancer.

When you choose the recommended chocolate with nuts, you'll also benefit from the almonds. In a study done at the University of California–Davis, researchers determined that almond consumption may provide some protection against the development of colon cancer in rats. Researchers believe that colon cancer is a diet-based disease, and a diet high in fiber (which is present in almonds) helps reduce the possibility of developing this type of cancer.

Add the dark chocolate–covered orange peel, and you'll benefit from the vitamin C in this nutrient-rich fruit. The role of vitamin C in combating cancer has long been established. In fact, one study tracked results from twenty-three centers in ten European countries, confirming that as little as 160 milligrams of vitamin C helped protect against stomach and esophagus cancers.

Cataracts

Recommendation

Take 4 squares dark chocolate with fresh or dried blueberries, twice daily as needed, with a maximum 12 squares in a single day. Wear glasses as required by your ophthalmologist.

Supporting Evidence

As certain people age, cataracts develop, the result of proteins that no longer function properly. As these proteins break down, they clump together to form cataracts, thus clouding the lens of the eye. Cataracts deflect light entering the eye and compromise the eye's ability create a clear image.

A number of studies have established that people who consume higher levels of antioxidant-rich foods have significantly fewer cataracts and less cases of macular degeneration. As you learned in chapter 3, and throughout the book, both blueberries and chocolate are very high in antioxidants, which is why they're in this particular recommendation.

Blueberries also contain vitamin C. According to a report published in the *American Journal of Clinical Nutrition*, subjects who took high concentrations (1 gram or more) of vitamin C daily showed significantly lower levels of cataracts than the control group did.

Another comprehensive ten-year report called the Blue Mountains Eye Study confirmed that protein, vitamin A, thiamine, niacin, and riboflavin all protect eyes from cataract damage. Chocolate contains trace amounts of each of these nutrients. The same study also found that smoking and high alcohol consumption correlated with a higher percentage of cataracts. So if you want a clearer picture, toss out the cigs and the martinis, and grab a dark chocolate bar, a bowl of blueberries, and a glass of red wine.

Cavities

Recommendation

Take 1 ounce 70% dark chocolate after meals and prior to brushing your teeth. Eat an apple afterward to help clean your teeth. Smile.

Supporting Evidence

Although dark chocolate is made with some sugar, it also contains phosphates, minerals, and other plant compounds that inhibit the growth of bacteria that promote tooth decay. In his book *The Cacahuatl Eater: Ruminations of an Unabashed Chocolate Addict*, author Jonathon Ott cites theobromine as the primary component of chocolate that helps fend off tooth decay.

The Eastman Dental Center in Rochester, New York, agrees that "chocolate is one of the snack foods least likely to contribute to tooth decay." Another interesting study from the *Journal of Indian Society of Pedodontics & Preventive Dentistry* showed that children who rinsed with a formula of chocolate mouthwash had 20 percent less plaque buildup than the control group had. As usual, eat dark chocolate, as opposed to milk chocolate, to get more minerals and less sugar.

Chronic Fatigue

Recommendation

In the morning: replace coffee with 1 cup hot cocoa made exactly as recommended in chapter 9. For dessert: ½ bar dark chocolate with goji berries, cinnamon, and almonds.

Supporting Evidence

Chronic diseases are on the rampage, and the statistics are shocking—approximately 60 percent of women and 40 percent of men over the age of sixty-five suffer from some type of chronic degeneration. Although chronic fatigue is not as acute as heart disease, cancer, obesity, and diabetes, it can be extremely debilitating to sufferers. Some people experience symptoms for years and even decades. It can also cause the onset of other very significant problems, such as depression and insomnia.

The exact cause of chronic fatigue is not known. Effects and intensity vary significantly from person to person, making the cause even more difficult to pinpoint. Many doctors simply write prescriptions to overcome the onslaught of symptoms. But speak to an educated dietician, and your prescription is likely to include a significant amount of antioxidant-rich foods.

It's no coincidence that disease increases concurrently with a higher consumption of processed, sugary, overcooked, and fatty foods. Experts agree that nutritious foods are crucial for optimal health, and studies support the consensus by showing that people who include whole fruits and vegetables in their daily diet have lower rates of almost all diseases. Enter chocolate.

As you know by now, chocolate is very rich in antioxidants. Antioxidants help rejuvenate cells, boost the immune system, increase blood flow, fight free radicals, and rid the body of poisonous toxins. Chocolate contains a variety of antioxidants that are readily absorbed by the body. Researchers from the United Kingdom clearly consolidated the concept in their report titled "High Cocoa Polyphenol Rich Chocolate Improves the Symptoms of Chronic Fatigue." That's straight to the point.

People who add the goji berries, as recommended, will get even more antioxidants from the superpowerful berries. Goji berries boast one of the highest levels of antioxidants of any berry on the planet. The recommended dose of cinnamon promotes better glucose metabolism, helping to keep blood sugar and energy levels stable.

Constipation

Recommendation

Almond bark: Microwave 1 dark chocolate bar in a glass bowl for 30 seconds on low power. Stir, then microwave for an additional 30 seconds. Repeat at 30-second intervals on low heat until the chocolate is melted. Mix in 10–20 almonds, stir, and refrigerate for 15 minutes. Take ¼ bar every hour with hot water and lemon juice until the problem is alleviated, not to exceed 1 bar of chocolate in a 24-hour period.

Supporting Evidence

One hundred grams of dark chocolate contain up to 10 grams of fiber, a substance known for its ability to help the body eliminate waste. Certain plant chemicals in chocolate also stimulate contractions of the intestinal canal. Even the Aztec and Maya civilizations recognized chocolate's ability to get things moving. Ancient journals repeatedly confirm that one of the top three medicinal uses of cocoa was kidney and bowel stimulation.

One reason chocolate helps with elimination is that it's a rich source of magnesium, a mineral that is especially good for the digestive system. It relaxes both the small and the large intestine. Once they're relaxed, digested food begins to move more smoothly, and this can be very helpful for constipation. This explains the name of Milk of Magnesia, which, of course, is made with magnesium.

Follow the recommendation by adding a healthy dose of almonds to the chocolate. According to the California Almond Board, eating almonds helps maintain the overall health of the gastrointestinal tract (www.AlmondBoard.com). One ounce of almonds contains 3 grams of fiber. With this in mind, the prescription calls for a chocolate/almond nut bark for the highest level of benefits.

Drinking a hot beverage with an alkaline-inducing infusion such as lemon juice may be helpful as well. Many people report that drinking coffee helps with the task at hand, but coffee (caffeine) is a diuretic that causes the body to lose water. It's estimated that 75 percent of us are dehydrated at any given time, and, in fact, dehydration is a major cause of constipation for the population at large. Drinking hot water with natural cleansers such as lemon or lime juice is better than a caffeinated beverage. Lemon juice also helps rebalance the body and bring blood pH levels back to normal—more factors that can assist with constipation.

Cough

Recommendation

One serving hot chocolate, made as directed in chapter 9. Take as needed, with a bowl of chicken soup, if preferred. Refrain from working or going to school, if applicable, for at least 1 day.

Supporting Evidence

Coughing is caused by the aggravation of sensitive nerve endings in the lung and bronchial areas of the body. It can be brought on by triggers such as pollen, pet dander, or cigarette smoke. Coughing can also be a side effect of having a cold. Dozens of cough medicines are on the market, but the high alcohol content and morphinelike suppressants in many cough medicines may have people looking outside the pharmacy for a healthier remedy.

Theobromine is the substance in chocolate that can help alleviate coughing. In 2005, the National Heart and Lung Institute in London conducted a study that compared theobromine to codeine (a popular ingredient in cough medicine) for its effectiveness in suppressing coughs. In this double-blind study, theobromine proved to be equally as effective as codeine. The study also pointed out that the two most widely distributed cough suppressants—codeine and dextromethorphan—are both opioid derivatives that frequently carry numerous adverse side effects. Theobromine showed no such side effects.

Although the amount of theobromine in a serving of chocolate is quite minimal compared to a dose of cough syrup, it still offers some benefits. Because of its antioxidants and other wonderful, euphoric-inducing components, homemade chocolate milk is an excellent choice when nursing a cough.

Some research suggests that adding dairy products to chocolate decreases its antioxidant benefits. Many people are also allergic to cow's milk, often without even realizing it. This condition induces more coughing and congestion. To make certain that you obtain the maximum amount of antioxidants from your hot cocoa, you may want to consider substituting rice, almond, or soy milk for regular cow's milk. Both rice and soy milk contain an estimated 30 percent of the daily requirement for calcium.

Cramps

Recommendation

Take 2 ounces melted dark chocolate with fresh sliced apples, fresh berries, cherries, and sunflower seeds. See "How to Microwave Chocolate" in chapter 9, because you'll need to mix up your own prescription.

Supporting Evidence

Cramps occur for a wide variety of reasons. Regardless of why they arrive, we're usually in a mad rush to find remedies to get rid of them. A quick overstatement of the obvious: if chocolate caused your cramps, eating more chocolate won't help them go away. The above recommendation is for everyone else.

Note that this recommendation is for dark chocolate, which doesn't contain lactose. As mentioned in "Cough," earlier, lactose is an enzyme that many people are unable to digest. In fact, it's estimated that fifty million people are lactose intolerant, and many of them don't even realize it. If you're not able to digest lactose and you eat milk chocolate, cramps will likely be one side effect.

An estimated 50 percent of us have taken antacids for cramps and indigestion. Yet nutrition experts agree that in the long run, an increase in antioxidants, rather than antacids, will likely offer the most relief. A diet high in antioxidant-rich foods helps keep the body running smoothly on all levels, including digestion.

As you've seen throughout this book, chocolate contains one of the highest levels of antioxidants of any food, provided that you focus on brands with good-quality ingredients and higher percentages of cocoa. (See "Wrapper Reading 101" in chapter 4 to get the most punch for your penny.)

Fresh fruits and seeds are included in the recommendation because these foods are known therapeutic digestive aids. Cramps are generally caused by indigestion, so foods that alleviate this condition are obviously ideal. Other digestive aids on the list include chocolate-friendly foods such as pomegranate, sesame seeds, currants, cherries, and bananas. Also on the list but not quite as good when paired with chocolate are cabbage, radishes, green beans, and spinach.

If your cramps have arrived concurrent with your "time of the month," make sure to read the sections on "PMS" and "Stress." Although chocolate probably won't relieve this particular discomfort, it's bound to make you feel better.

Depression

Recommendation

Take 4 squares dark chocolate with dried fruit every hour as needed, not to exceed a maximum of 1.75 ounces in any 24-hour period. Read an uplifting novel, and repeat positive affirmations between doses.

Supporting Evidence

Chocolate helps stimulate the secretion of several endorphins that are beneficial to a state of well-being. One of these is tryptophan, an amino acid that creates mood-enhancing effects. Tryptophan is the precursor to the feel-good chemical serotonin, a primary neurotransmitter that helps reduce anxiety and keep stress under control. Chocolate also contains phenylethylamine (PEA), which causes the body to release dopamine, another neurotransmitter known for its mood-enhancing and relaxation effects.

One study even stated that eating chocolate may produce the same pleasurable sensation as running several miles, but after a brief poll, I discovered that most people would opt for the chocolate. Perhaps it would be wise to do both, particularly if you discover you've exceeded the recommended daily dosage.

If you follow the recommendation exactly, you'll benefit from the dried fruit as well. Studies comparing various populations have concluded that eating fruit may reduce the possibility of developing a host of problems, including diabetes, cataracts, heart failure, indigestion, PMS, and strokes. Although none of these ailments is specifically depression, avoiding them by eating healthier foods will give you considerably fewer reasons to be depressed.

A note on positive affirmations: make sure they're positive! Affirmations should be free of negative words.

Not acceptable: I won't eat more than the recommended amount of chocolate for my condition.

Acceptable: I easily keep my chocolate consumptions at a healthy level.

Diabetes

Recommendation

Take 1 small piece low-glycemic chocolate 3 times daily, once at each meal, with 5 mixed nuts (unless nuts are included in the chocolate).

Supporting Evidence

Diabetes is a condition of having perpetually high blood sugar, a state that is toxic to the body. When people eat high-glycemic foods (typically, processed foods, carbs, and sweets), the body releases insulin into the bloodstream to lower the blood sugar. Diabetics have lost the ability to manufacture insulin on their own, so they need to monitor their diets to keep their blood sugar from spiking. That means eating "low glycemic index" foods.

The glycemic index is a 0–100 scale that rates foods on how they affect blood sugar. Foods made of refined grains and refined sugar, such as cookies, cakes, and sugary candies, all rate high on the index (60+), meaning that they raise blood sugar when they're eaten. Healthier foods, such as whole grains, fresh fruits and vegetables, nuts, and meats, rank lower. (See appendix B for a complete review of this subject.) Chocolate makes the low-glycemic cut because it comes in at 50 on the glycemic index. If you eat it with the recommended nuts, however, it comes in at a very low 33.

It's estimated that by the year 2015, 75 percent of the people in the United States will be overweight. Unfortunately, weight gain is often associated with the onset of type 2 diabetes. Once the disease sets in, compounding health problems begin to occur, such as heart disease, dementia, arthritis, and more. In December 2008, *Prevention Magazine* released a special issue called "Outsmart Diabetes." The feature article listed on the front page was "Reverse Diabetes with Food." Proper eating can not only prevent type 2 diabetes from occurring, but it can also reverse the process once it is in motion.

Education is the key to healthy chocolate enjoyment, and this especially holds true for diabetics. Even the American College of Cardiology reported in 2008 that dark chocolate consumption can help reverse vascular dysfunction in diabetics.

Here are the basic guidelines for diabetics and chocolate:

Eat 70%+ dark chocolate. Look for the percentage on the outside of the wrapper.

Eat chocolate with nuts. The protein, fat, and fiber in nuts help slow the absorption of food into the bloodstream, keeping the blood sugar lower. Nuts also contain vitamin E, an antioxidant that has been shown to help metabolize glucose in diabetic patients.

Read the labels. Avoid butterfat, milk fat, and other added fats (with the exception of cocoa butter). Artificial flavors and sweeteners should also be avoided.

Look for chocolates sweetened with evaporated cane juice or agave nectar—both are lower-glycemic sweeteners than processed white sugar. An example is Xocai chocolate, which is diabetic friendly. It also doesn't contain any caffeine or artificial sweeteners and has added blueberry and acai berry powder (available at www.TheChocolateTherapist .com/buyxocai.php).

Doggy Danger

Recommendation

No chocolate of any kind for dogs—ever!

Supporting Evidence

Dogs should never eat chocolate because they lack the enzyme to metabolize theobromine, one of the stimulants in chocolate. This makes it impossible for dogs to remove theobromine from their system. The dog's heart speeds up, and it can literally have a heart attack. Dogs don't have to eat much chocolate for their reaction to become a serious medical emergency. A toxic dose for a fifty-pound dog can be as small as 5 ounces of baking chocolate, an amount a dog can snap up in a couple of seconds.

The severity of the reaction varies with the type of chocolate. Milk chocolate is at least 50% sugar and doesn't contain as much theobromine, so some dogs can tolerate milk chocolate without issue. But dark chocolate contains considerably more theobromine, so, of course, it's much more toxic to dogs. If your dog eats a bar of dark chocolate, call the vet immediately.

Another thing to be aware of is cocoa mulch for the yard, which works wonderfully if you don't have dogs. According to the statistics from one manufacturer, 98 percent of dogs won't eat the mulch. Of the 2 percent that do, only half of them have severe reactions, which include vomiting, a racing heart, and sometimes death. This means that one in a hundred dogs has a chance of having severe reactions or dying if it eats cocoa mulch.

The problem is easily solved: if you have dogs, don't put cocoa mulch on your yard. You can also look for theobromine-free cocoa mulch, now available as manufacturers seek to address this issue.

Emphysema

Recommendation

Take 3 squares 70%+ caffeine-free dark chocolate in the mid-morning and midafternoon. Stop smoking (if you do), begin an exercise program, avoid allergens, and eat small meals frequently.

Supporting Evidence

Emphysema is a lung disease that greatly hinders the lungs' ability to function properly. Sufferers experience a reduced capacity to breathe and may even require the aid of oxygen tanks. Unfortunately, the disease is considered irreversible, so once you have it, you're likely to feel worse as time progresses. It hardly seems like a bar of chocolate would offer much relief, but read on.

Chocolate stimulates the body to release nitric oxide, a compound that helps dilate bloods vessels up to 20 percent. This increases blood flow allowing the arteries to deliver more blood to the body, and blood contains oxygen and nutrients. People suffering from emphysema have less oxygen in the blood, so greater blood flow can combat this issue.

A number of dietary strategies can also be implemented to improve breathing. According to www.EHealthMD.com, people who suffer from emphysema should avoid caffeine, and, fortunately, there's not much caffeine in chocolate. As you've seen a number of times in various remedies, a typical 2-ounce bar has less caffeine than a cup of decaf coffee. This means it's better to avoid coffee, rather than chocolate, if you're trying to cut down on caffeine.

If you can't bear the thought of sacrificing your morning cup, consider replacing it with brewing cocoa, a new product from Choffy (available at www.TheChocolateTherapist.com/Choffy .php). It tastes very similar to coffee, brews in the coffeepot, doesn't contain sugar, and has 75 percent less caffeine than a cup of decaf (0–5 milligrams per cup). It's made from ground cocoa beans instead of coffee beans. You get a mild stimulant effect from the theobromine without experiencing the upset stomach that caffeine can sometimes cause. Brewing cocoa contains all of the antioxidant benefits of chocolate and almost no calories—it's certainly worth a try!

Another dietary strategy for people suffering from emphysema is eating many small meals throughout the day—hence the recommendation to eat chocolate between meals, rather than at a meal. A full stomach can make breathing more difficult, so it's best to keep your meals small.

Overall, emphysema is a very difficult disease to live with, because you can feel as if you're in a continual state of semi-suffocation. Your anxiety and stress will obviously be high, and chocolate can help here as well. In addition to the physical benefits mentioned earlier, chocolate offers a cocktail of psychological advantages, because it contains substances that cause the body to release endorphins and other stress-relieving neurotransmitters.

Energy Loss

Recommendation

Take 2 squares dark chocolate with dried berries or other dried fruit after lunch, every 2 hours until dinnertime. After eating the chocolate, take 10 deep breaths and hold for 4 seconds each, then exhale. Do not exceed a maximum of 12 squares in a 24-hour period.

Supporting Evidence

The case for chocolate as an energy source lands on both sides of the fence. On one hand, chocolate contains carbohydrates and sugar that the body quickly absorbs to convert into energy. Yet it also contains fat, which slows the absorption of sugars into the blood. Picking up your energy level requires a quick infusion of foods that raise blood sugar, but preferably these will be healthy food choices, as opposed to processed sugar. So, when attempting to increase your energy levels, consider chocolate *and* its added ingredients to get the job done. Dried fruit is an excellent choice.

An estimated six pounds of fresh fruit creates only one pound of dried fruit, and caloric and vitamin value are fully retained. The body readily absorbs the sugars in fruit, both glucose and fructose, making them an ideal choice for replenishing energy reserves.

Chocolate's high magnesium content also benefits people who want to increase their energy. You'll see magnesium referenced throughout the book because it's abundant in chocolate. Magnesium helps activate dozens of enzymes that manufacture and transport energy, a key component in keeping energy levels up. Because all of the magnesium in chocolate is in the cocoa powder, darker is better, as usual.

The central nervous system stimulants caffeine and theobromine are back in the picture as well. Although the amount of the two compounds is relatively small, here's the readers-only secret to gaining maximum energy for the effort: eat chocolate-covered cocoa nibs—however, they're guaranteed to keep you up all night if you eat enough of them before bedtime (available at www.TheChocolateTherapist.com/buycacao.com). See how they perform double duty if your diet lacks fiber (coming up next).

Fiber Shortage

Recommendation

Take 3 tablespoons chocolate-covered cocoa nibs in the morning to help get things moving. Optional: regular cocoa nibs without the chocolate.

Supporting Evidence

It's highly unlikely that you've seen chocolate at the top of the list of fiber-rich foods. After all, a 100-gram bar of 70% dark chocolate contains only 6–10 grams of fiber, and it has to be top-quality chocolate to have that much. Most bars have considerably less. In fact, if you were relying on chocolate alone, you'd need to eat at least a pound of chocolate per day to reach the average 25-gram minimum fiber requirement (your total fiber requirement varies, depending on your age, sex, weight, and activity level).

But not to worry! Chocolate-covered cocoa nibs are the answer to this problem, along with being a rich source of anti-oxidants and nutrients. By weight, cocoa nibs are approximately 9 percent fiber, 12 percent protein, and 20 percent polyphenols (after fermentation). If you read "Energy Loss" just prior to this section, you'll realize that chocolate gives you the double benefit of an energy boost along with your dose of fiber.

Fibromyalgia

Recommendation

Don't eat chocolate—not dark or milk or white, with nuts or without, with spices or without, with dried fruits or without. Just say no. But read this entire section anyway, especially if you can't imagine the thought of giving up your love (chocolate, not your significant other!).

Supporting Evidence

Nearly 100 percent of the research advises against eating chocolate if you suffer from fibromyalgia, a syndrome characterized by chronic muscle pain and relentless exhaustion. Dietary recommendations include much of what we'd expect to see from any good diet—focus on whole fresh foods, eat fewer processed and sugary foods, balance your blood sugar, get enough sleep, and drink plenty of pure water.

Interestingly, one key recommendation to combat fibromyalgia is eating antioxidant-rich foods to help build the immune system. A few more crucial bits of advice—avoid caffeine and sugar-laden desserts, eat small meals throughout the day, remove artificial ingredients from your diet, and eat organic foods.

It's my observation that a serving of freshly sliced organic fruits dipped in melted 70% dark organic chocolate spiced with ground ginger qualifies as a whole, nonprocessed food choice that helps keep blood sugar low, just what the experts advise. It's certainly worth considering. If you don't know where you can find this unique concoction, visit www.TheChocolateTherapist

.com and e-mail your request. We'll custom-create a chocolate for you. You can also read "How to Microwave Chocolate" in chapter 9 in order to make your own home brew.

Sufferers might note that more than 50 percent of people with fibromyalgia have vitamin D deficiencies. Fish and fish oils are some of the richest sources of this vitamin, but ask your doctor about taking extra supplementation.

Flatulence

Recommendation

Take ½ bar (1 ounce) dark chocolate with mint. Drink 1 cup mint tea, and take 4 peppermint breath mints, if needed, for emergency situations.

Supporting Evidence

Chocolate was used as medicine long before it became a delicacy sweetened with sugar, spices, and milk. Centuries ago, one of its most prevalent uses was as a digestive aid. When you combine chocolate with mint, another centuries-old digestive aid, you get just the right combination for quick relief. Mint is a stimulant that counteracts spasms in the digestive tract. It promotes the release of bile and gastric secretions as well, adding to the overall digestive flow. Be sure to follow the entire recommendation for an increased level of comfort, especially prior to a business meeting.

Note: do *not* use sugar-free chocolate for this recommendation, because artificial sweeteners have been shown to cause indigestion, as well as act as a laxative. In fact, "indigestion" is a mild understatement because if you eat a single 2-ounce sugar-free chocolate bar containing maltitol before a meeting, you'll probably be looking for more than one excuse to leave the room within an hour. There's no reason to eat sugar-free candy, although it's becoming more popular as diabetes spreads in epidemic proportions. Two words of wisdom: consumer beware.

Food Cravings

Recommendation

Take 1 square milk chocolate, 1 square dark chocolate, and 1 cup hot cocoa made with real cocoa (see the recipe in chapter 9). Repeat as needed until cravings subside, up to a maximum of 1 ounce chocolate per day.

Supporting Evidence

This is hardly a surprising statistic: more than half of all food cravings are said to involve chocolate. Another "astounding" fact: chocolate is the number one food that women crave. And of those who declared chocolate to be their top craving, 75 percent stated that *only* chocolate would curb their craving. In other words, denying a craving or trying to curb it by eating something else isn't likely to work. It's better to cave in to a craving and not feel guilty about it than it is to eat hundreds of additional calories trying to deny it.

Consider this example: if you eat 500 calories' worth of sugar-free cookies and low-carb chips but still want chocolate, you're over the limit by 500 calories and still left with the original craving. According to Debra Waterhouse, the author of *Why Women Need Chocolate*, a chocolate craving can be satisfied by consuming just one Hershey's Kiss (25 calories). Even a 10-Kiss/250-calorie splurge is better than binging on everything in sight, while you try to ignore a craving. Debra uses Hershey's Kisses in her book, but it would be better to enjoy a 70% dark chocolate square for maximum benefit.

Chocolate's perfectly balanced blend of sugar and fat also uniquely satisfies food cravings. The body contains an amino acid peptide called galanin that stimulates the appetite. Galanin is shut off by fats, which help trigger satiation. Because chocolate contains fat, it helps curb the effect of galanin, lessening the desire to eat. People also biologically crave fat when endorphins are low. Consumption of chocolate stimulates the release of both endorphins and serotonin into the brain. Endorphins transmit energy and feelings of euphoria, and serotonin evokes calmness and mood stability.

Here's another unique twist to cravings: if you talk about eating chocolate before you do it, you're likely to eat less. In a study performed at the University of Hertfordshire on chocolate and food behavior, researchers discovered that when people talk about chocolate after thinking about consuming it, they're likely to eat less than if they repress their thoughts. The results were particularly true for women. Those who didn't discuss their thoughts ate considerably more chocolate than those who did. The researchers concluded that verbal repression resulted in more chocolate consumption.

Cocoa also contains more than four hundred distinct flavor compounds. It's conceivable that by eating only one little piece of chocolate, many of your extraneous cravings can be contained. The moral of the story: When addressing cravings, go right to the source of the problem and simply have a piece of chocolate. Attempting to deny the craving may cause you to consume every morsel of food within a six-mile radius. Follow the recommendation and end the craving before monumental damage is done.

Going to the Dark Side

This is for those who need assistance in converting from milk to dark chocolate.

Recommendation

Eat 1 square basic milk chocolate, followed directly by 1 square high-quality milk chocolate, followed directly by 1 square of high-quality dark chocolate. Use the guidelines in chapter 5 to ensure maximum effectiveness, and rinse with a full-bodied cabernet sauvignon between chocolates (water is also acceptable). Take this remedy after the lunchtime or evening meal.

Supporting Evidence

Although it tastes delicious, milk chocolate is not the ideal choice for people who want to obtain health benefits from chocolate. It contains far too many fats and sugars. Milk chocolate is like fried zucchini—the initial food in its raw form is wonderful, but by the time the cooked item reaches your mouth, it's so heavily disguised that it's virtually unrecognizable. Follow this simple procedure to acquire a true appreciation for the darker delicacy.

The best way to accomplish the task is to host a "vertical pairing" for yourself and your significant other (in the absence of such a person, children or neighbors work perfectly as substitutes). Purchase a generic milk chocolate, a high-quality milk chocolate, a semisweet chocolate (about 45% dark), and a bittersweet chocolate (about 60–65% dark). Line them up with a bland cracker in between each chocolate. Start by eating the lightest chocolate and move to the darkest, taking time to enjoy the flavors as each chocolate melts in your mouth. Cleanse your palate with a cracker and water or wine in between. (You don't need to devour four entire bars; this is where the significant others come in— they will save you from having to hit the gym for twenty-four hours after you're finished.)

Once you've eaten a sample of each, try going back to the milk chocolate. Do this right after eating the darkest chocolate so that you can see just how sweet the milk chocolate is. You won't really be able to taste the flavors in the milk chocolate because they're buried in sugar.

The process may take a little practice before you can officially make the switch: a little milk, a little dark, a little milk, a little dark. You'll know whether you've advanced to proper chocolate-for-health snobbery when you truly enjoy dark chocolate.

Headache

Recommendation

Take ½ ounce dark chocolate with a freshly sliced apple and a sprinkle of sea salt. Consume these directly after a meal. Lie down for 10 minutes afterward, elevate your feet, and breathe deeply.

Supporting Evidence

A number of people claim that chocolate causes their migraines, but others say it's the only thing that stops them. How can both statements be true?

Some headaches are caused by a rush of blood to the head; others by a lack of it. How chocolate affects your headache depends on which type of headache you suffer from. If yours is caused by lack of blood, chocolate may help you. Eating dark chocolate raises the level of nitric oxide in the blood, a chemical compound that dilates blood vessels and allows more blood to pass through them. Aspirin works in much the same way in the brain by expanding constricted blood vessels, allowing more blood to flow through and reducing pain.

But do you have to eat ten chocolate bars to benefit? According to a study done at a University of California nutrition department, eating only 25 grams of semisweet chocolate has a similar effect on the body as consuming an 81-milligram dose of aspirin.

If you suffer from headaches caused by a rush of blood to the head, as in migraines, chocolate won't help. As mentioned earlier, eating chocolate helps dilate blood vessels, and some migraines are caused by a rush of blood to the head. Yet it's still possible that something else and not the cocoa is the actual cause of the headaches.

In a double-blind study at the University of Pittsburgh, subjects were given chocolate and carob (a food that tastes like chocolate but doesn't contain cocoa) over a two-week period. The results demonstrated little difference in chocolate and carob as migraine triggers. In fact, the researchers determined that chocolate does not appear to trigger headaches. More than one study has come to this same conclusion.

A high-quality 70% dark chocolate bar with healthy ingredients such as cocoa powder, cocoa butter, and evaporated cane juice is your best choice because it contains more cocoa and less sugar. Migraine sufferers might also want to read *The Miracle of Magnesium* by Dr. Carolyn Dean. It contains very specific information on the benefits of magnesium for migraines. A few hundred milligrams of magnesium per day could be the secret ingredient that cures your headaches.

Final food for thought: if you know that chocolate triggers your headache, you're one of those whom it affects negatively. Just say no.

Heartbreak

Recommendation

Unlimited extremely dark chocolate squares (such as baking chocolate) as needed. Call friends in the morning. Avoid sappy movies about lovers, sad or melancholy music, depressing books, and rain.

Supporting Evidence

Admittedly, a recommendation to eat baking chocolate is extreme. But a broken heart calls for drastic measures, and the darker the better. Chocolate contains a powerful amphetamine called phenylethylamine (PEA). Although the amount of PEA is relatively small, its effects on the brain are measurable after the consumption of chocolate. PEA triggers a release of natural opiatelike chemicals that induce feelings of bliss. PEA is also the same chemical the brain emits when you experience the rush of falling in love. And not surprisingly, there's even a substantial increase of PEA during orgasm.

Chocolate offers up quite a collection of positives—natural opiatelike compounds, the feeling of falling in love, and orgasmic bliss. Clearly, it satisfies at least a few of our basic love needs without our having to suffer through the arguments or the frustration of trying to navigate a challenging relationship. And at a trivial few dollars or less per bar, it's a superb value, when compared to $150 an hour or more for therapy. It's no mystery why it's a good idea to pamper a lovesick heart with a chocolate one.

Heart Disease

Recommendation

Take 8 squares dark chocolate with almonds and/or pomegranate for 3 days in a row after lunch, with one day off; repeat as needed, for life. Optional: exchange almonds for your nut of choice.

Supporting Evidence

Flavonoids are very powerful antioxidants found in fruits, vegetables, tea, and red wines. A subcategory of flavonoids called flavanols are similar health-enhancing compounds found in chocolate. Recent research shows that the antioxidant benefits of flavanols play a considerable role in preventing artery damage caused by free radicals. Flavanols have also been shown to help reduce platelet aggregation in the blood, decreasing the risk of having a heart attack or a stroke. Not long ago, red wine received a favorable nod as an excellent source of antioxidants. Yet a cup of hot chocolate made with pure cocoa contains almost twice as many antioxidants as a glass of red wine. (For maximum antioxidant effect, use soy, rice, or almond milk with the cocoa instead of dairy products, as was mentioned in chapter 4 in reference to studies at the University of Glasgow.)

Research on chocolate and its benefits for the heart is abundant. At the University of California, researchers fed 1.6 ounces of dark chocolate per day to twenty-two volunteers during the course of two weeks. Half of them received the actual chocolate and the other half a placebo. Those who received the chocolate showed significantly more relaxation in their blood vessels than those who didn't.

Another study from the University of Scranton in Pennsylvania reported multiple heart-health benefits from chocolate consumption, including "inhibited atherosclerosis, lowered cholesterol, raised high-density lipoproteins [good fats], and protection of lower density lipoproteins from oxidation." The study cited one of the antioxidants in chocolate called "epicatechin" as a "major inhibitor of plasma lipid oxidation." Oxidized lipids are bad for the body because they harden along the arteries' walls. Keeping them out of the system is crucial for optimal heart health.

Pomegranate is part of the recommendation because it also offers major benefits for the heart. In fact, you'll see pomegranate included under "High Blood Pressure," further on. One study demonstrated that people who drank 8 ounces of pomegranate juice daily for three months experienced a 17 percent increase in blood flow to the heart. Participants in the placebo group actually had reduced flow to their hearts. Pomegranate not only brings a powerful boost to the heart, but it tastes wonderful with chocolate as well.

Adding nuts to chocolate, as recommended, also strengthens the heart. Nuts are high in monounsaturated and polyunsaturated fats, both of which are considered healthy fats. Consuming nuts has actually been linked to a decrease in risk for heart attacks. A recent study at Tufts University in Boston found that a phyto-chemical (plant compound) contained in the skin of almonds, combined with the vitamin E in the almond itself, protected LDL cholesterol ("bad fats") from oxidation. Eating nuts has also been shown to increase HDL cholesterol ("good fats") in the bloodstream. The net result is more good fats and fewer bad fats.

High Blood Pressure / Hypertension

Recommendation

Take 4–6 squares dark chocolate with macadamia nuts after dinner with a glass of red wine. Listen to baroque-style music (60 beats per minute or slower) with both feet propped up on the couch for a minimum of 10 minutes before proceeding with your evening plans.

Supporting Evidence

Salt and high blood pressure have a cause-and-effect relationship that has been around for years. Yet a study done on the Kuna people, a tribe living off the coast of Panama, discovered that despite their having a high-salt diet, their blood pressure levels were extremely low. The chocolate connection? The Kuna drink about five cups of chocolate per day. A follow-up study done at Harvard University confirmed the possible link. Volunteers were fed both milk chocolate and dark chocolate. Those who consumed the equivalent amount of dark chocolate as the Kuna people showed a marked increase in nitric oxide in their blood. Nitric oxide helps dilate blood vessels, reducing blood pressure by allowing more blood to pass through them.

A Greek study produced similar results when testing participants' artery relaxation. After fasting for five hours, half of the group received 100 grams of chocolate (3.5-ounce bar) for a snack and the other half received nothing. The researchers tested both blood flow and pulse for three hours by ultrasound. The chocolate consumers' arteries dilated 20 percent more than did the arteries of those who had not eaten chocolate. The highest dilation occurred after three hours (the end of the test), suggesting that the benefits continued to increase even after the test was over.

To get similar blood pressure–reducing results yourself, you must eat chocolate with a high percentage of cocoa (70+%). One study showed that people who were given a beverage containing low levels of cocoa flavanols showed no relaxation in blood vessels, while those given high levels of cocoa flavanols had positive results.

More good news for magnesium as well: researchers have discovered a link between hypertension and a deficiency in magnesium. As mentioned earlier, cocoa is one of the highest natural sources of magnesium of all foods. Meeting the daily magnesium requirement has proved to be beneficial for both the cardiovascular system and hypertension. A 3-ounce bar contains 115 milligrams of magnesium, approximately 25 percent of the daily magnesium requirement.

If you choose a chocolate with macadamia nuts, as suggested, you'll benefit even more. Macadamia nuts are high in monounsaturated "good fats," which help lower cholesterol.

High Cholesterol

Recommendation

Take ½ bar 60% dark chocolate with nuts, sesame seeds, and/ or pomegranate daily with your afternoon tea and a selection of fresh fruit. Caution: reading the labels is imperative—eat only chocolate with cocoa butter and no other fats.

Supporting Evidence

Some doctors advise patients against eating chocolate to avoid high cholesterol, and for good reason: much of the chocolate consumed today is in fact cause for alarm. Some chocolates list hydrogenated oils, milk fat, vegetable oil, and sugar as their main ingredients, all of which are villains in the war against bad cholesterol. A quick label-reading lesson (see "Wrapper Reading 101" in chapter 4) and a little knowledge about cholesterol can help set the record straight.

Contrary to popular belief, cutting out dietary cholesterol is not the be-all and end-all of reducing your actual cholesterol count. According to author Mary Enig (*Know Your Fats*), 70 to 80 percent of the cholesterol in your body is actually manufactured by your cells. All of the fuss about lowering dietary cholesterol doesn't help many people at all. After forgoing foods they love for years, they still end up taking cholesterol-reducing medications for their chronic high cholesterol. One of the best strategies is to eat foods that are rich in antioxidants because these remove excess cholesterol from the bloodstream. Good-quality dark chocolate is one of these foods. "Bad" LDL cholesterol clogs the arteries, while "good" HDL helps clean them. Eating dark chocolate on a regular basis has been shown to lower LDL and raise HDL, exactly what you'd like to see for optimal cholesterol health.

At the University of Pennsylvania, a study compared subjects who were given cocoa butter with another group that was given regular butter. People who were fed cocoa butter showed no increase in cholesterol levels, while those who were given regular butter showed an increase.

In another study conducted at Pennsylvania State University, researchers instructed a group of volunteers to add 16 grams of dark chocolate and 22 grams of cocoa powder to their daily diet. As a result, all of the volunteers experienced improved cholesterol levels. Even the LDL cholesterol appeared to be more resistant to oxidation by free radicals, making it less dangerous to the heart.

In a similar study, researchers gave volunteers a milk chocolate bar for a snack instead of a high-carbohydrate alternative (bagel, chips, etc.). The subjects' level of HDL increased, while the bad cholesterol remained unchanged, suggesting that your cholesterol levels can improve if you eat chocolate. Had the researchers used high-quality dark chocolate, the results would have been even more impressive.

Although it's true that chocolate contains fat, most of it is cholesterol friendly. A 2-ounce dark chocolate bar contains approximately 11 grams of fat, more than half of it saturated. Yet a quick education about fats can put your mind at ease, because "saturated" doesn't always mean "bad." Approximately 35–41 percent of the fat in dark chocolate is oleic acid—the same fat that is found in olive oil and that has been shown to have a slight cholesterol-lowering effect. About 34–39 percent of the fat is stearic acid, which is unique compared to other saturated fats because it does not raise blood cholesterol levels. Only 23–30 percent of the fat in chocolate is palmitic acid, which is considered a "bad fat." The final 5 percent is linoleic acid, an essential fatty acid and an extremely important substance in your overall health regimen.

Chocolate with pomegranate is part of the recommendation, because research has shown this fruit to be highly effective in reducing oxidative damage related to high cholesterol. A study reported in *Clinical Nutrition* showed that people who consumed pomegranate juice daily had less thickening of the arteries. In addition, their cholesterol oxidation rate was reduced by nearly 50 percent.

Sesame seeds can also provide benefits in cholesterol reduction, hence the recommendation to include them with your chocolate. According to a study in the *Journal of Nutrition*, women who took 3 tablespoons of sesame powder (made from ground sesame seeds) daily for three weeks experienced a 5 percent drop in total cholesterol and a 10 percent drop in LDL cholesterol. They also had more vitamin E in their blood and slower rates of LDL oxidation.

Finally, adding nuts to chocolate improves the body's HDL cholesterol count. Research has confirmed that people who eat nuts on a regular basis have significantly lower levels of heart disease. Almonds and walnuts are particularly healthful. In fact, some studies have shown that eating only one ounce of almonds per day can actually lower cholesterol levels. Yet even pistachios and hazelnuts have been reported to help lower cholesterol, so take your medicine!

Hyperglycemia / Hypoglycemia

Recommendation

Take 2 squares dark chocolate with dried berries or other dried fruit after lunch, every 2 hours until dinnertime. Do not exceed a maximum of 12 squares in a 24-hour period.

Supporting Evidence

Hyperglycemia is a condition of high blood sugar, and hypoglycemia is the opposite: low blood sugar. Hypoglycemia normally sets in first. When blood sugar drops, the brain is immediately affected because its basic fuel is glucose. It sends the alarm to eat something sweet to raise blood sugar levels back up. Unfortunately, most of us overshoot the mark, often indulging in something extraordinarily sweet that sends us into a state of hyperglycemia. When the postsugar crash ensues an hour later, you eat something else to lift you back up, conceivably keeping yourself on the seesaw all day long.

To prevent this from happening, the best strategy is to snack on low-glycemic foods such as nuts, certain fruits, cheeses, protein, and, fortunately, dark chocolate with nuts. These foods don't trigger an over-response from the body because they don't raise blood sugar excessively. To get a better understanding of low-glycemic foods and how they affect the body, review the "Diabetes" section earlier and appendix B as well. People who prefer to go all out with research will enjoy reading *The New Glucose Revolution Life Plan* by Jennie Brand-Miller.

Immune Deficiency

Recommendation

Take 3 squares dark chocolate and 1 cup hot cocoa made with real cocoa and the natural sweetener of your choice (see the recipe in chapter 9) when you feel an illness coming on. Optional: take 1,000 milligrams vitamin C as well.

Supporting Evidence

A study in Japan confirmed that chocolate contains phenolics, powerful compounds derived from plants that boosted the immune system when tested in human blood samples. Because they're a type of antioxidant, phenolics also have a proven ability to suppress body-damaging free radicals.

Yet immune-system support from chocolate doesn't end there. Dark chocolate contains a number of different types of antioxidants that are readily absorbed by the body. Of particular interest are catechin and epicatechin, both of which have been shown to help activate the body's natural detoxification process and promote a healthier immune system.

If you choose to follow the recommendation precisely, you'll also benefit from vitamin C, another immune system booster. The main sources of antioxidants are selenium, alpha lipoic acid, coenzyme Q10 (CoQ10), and the vitamins A, C, and E. Eat foods that are rich in nutrients, and you'll naturally consume an abundance of antioxidants.

For the Olympic-caliber antioxidant enthusiast, make up a batch of Chocolate Chocolate Chip Oatmeal Cookies (see the recipe in chapter 9) and throw in a handful of vitamin E–rich sunflower seeds and pecans. You'll have your own ultimate antioxidant cocktail with oats, seeds, nuts, and chocolate.

Impotence

Recommendation

Take 65% dark chocolate blended with walnuts, acai berries, and goji berries. Optional: l-arginine supplements once daily.

Supporting Evidence

Impotence has so many probable causes that it's impossible to isolate a single defining factor. This summary addresses physically based solutions through nutrition, although it's possible that a little chocolate consumption could also address a psychological issue or two.

Chocolate contains arginine, an amino acid that is often termed "nature's Viagra," due to its known blood-circulating effects. Arginine helps the body release nitric oxide into the blood, a compound that dilates blood vessels and allows more blood to circulate throughout the body. Of course, this includes crucial areas such as those affected by impotence. Arginine also plays a fundamental role in building the proteins of seminal fluid, so a deficiency can actually cause impotence (www.nutriherb.net/l-arginine.html). Nuts are part of the recommendation because they contain arginine, as do sesame seeds and sunflower seeds.

The recommendation includes the Amazonian acai and goji berries because, like chocolate, they're also proud recipients of the "nature's Viagra" nickname. These two berries contain some of the highest levels of antioxidants of any fruit on the planet, making them ideal partners when you're considering options for body repair. In the big picture, antioxidant-rich foods contain benefits for blood circulation, an obvious concern with impotence.

For true emergencies, of course, one chocolate bar won't take the place of a dose of Viagra, although Dr. Dora Akunyili might beg to differ. In an article titled "Viagra Works, but Chocolate Works Better," the doctor cites a Nigerian study that demonstrated chocolate's ability to stimulate the libido. Dr. Akunyili suggested taking pure cocoa powder in a pill form, but that's positively boring! Go with the chocolate concoction mentioned under "Recommendation." For significant longer-term results, you may want to add a dose of l-arginine to your daily diet, to avoid eating mountains of chocolate for the same effect. There's no U.S. Recommended Daily Allowance, but a typical supplement contains 500 milligrams per dose.

Infertility

Recommendation

Melt 2 ounces 65% dark chocolate in a microwave (see "How to Microwave Chocolate" in chapter 9). Dip dried apricot halves in the chocolate, place them on a plate, and refrigerate. Eat 2 after lunch every day.

Supporting Evidence

Just like impotence, infertility has so many probable causes that it takes a highly trained expert to successfully diagnose the issue. It's not surprising that as a nutritionist, I recommend a possible solution that involves nutrition, and chocolate is an excellent place to start.

The theme of this entire book is that chocolate is rich in antioxidants, a key element in fertility because antioxidants help build healthy cells, while clearing away toxins as well. As previously mentioned, antioxidants are present in vitamins A, C, E, and K; CoQ10; selenium; alpha lipoic acid; and a few other substances. Of these, vitamin C has been show to be particularly effective in treating impotence. A study from the *Proceedings of the National Academy of Sciences* showed that by reducing vitamin C from 250 milligrams a day to just 5 milligrams, sperm count was decreased an astounding 50 percent, with damaged sperm accounting for 91 percent of the total count. Conversely, men who were given 1,000 milligrams of vitamin C daily for one week showed a 140 percent increase in sperm count—in only *one* week!

I mention the vitamin C statistics here because the effects of these studies correspond to the vitamin's antioxidant qualities, and dark chocolate is very high in antioxidants. The recommended dried apricots are also high in vitamin C. Anything that protects and builds the body in one area will do the same thing everywhere. Antioxidants play an important role in sperm production, thus a shortage of antioxidants may contribute to a lowered sperm count.

Women can benefit from good-quality chocolate consumption for the same reasons—antioxidants rid the body of toxins and help build healthy cells for proper body functioning. Obviously, the issue is quite complex and requires a variety of strategies and adjustments to achieve success. To maximize antioxidant consumption, consume fresh and dried fruits, dark chocolate, green tea, and perhaps even an occasional glass of red wine.

Insomnia

Recommendation

Keep all chocolate consumption limited to the hours of 6:00 A.M. to 3:00 P.M. Absolutely no chocolate after 3:00 P.M., with the minor exception being that if you happen to desire ½ bar of 55% dark chocolate in the time period between 3:00 and 3:15 P.M., it may be consumed with 1–2 cups of chamomile tea.

Supporting Evidence

Insomnia is caused by many things, but professionals agree that one of the most predominant triggers is stress. Given the ever-changing economy, it's not surprising that the incidence of both stress and insomnia are significantly on the rise. Recommended dietary changes include not eating after 7:00 P.M., cutting down on extremely spicy food at the dinner meal, and staying away from caffeine after 4:00 P.M.

If you read "Caffeine Withdrawal" earlier, you're aware that chocolate doesn't contain much caffeine. In fact, there's less caffeine in a 2-ounce bar of chocolate than you'll get in a cup of decaf coffee. Many types of cocoa beans in the world have no caffeine at all, and more chocolates are becoming available without it (see www.TheChocolateTherapist.com/buyxocai.php).

But insomniacs take note—it's still in your best interest to keep chocolate on your do-not-consume-after-3:00-P.M. list. Chocolate contains a cocktail of stimulants, including theobromine and phenylethylamine. They're milder than caffeine but still cause the body to pick up and get ready for action.

Consuming chocolate also helps the body release nitric oxide, which can dilate blood vessels up to 20 percent. Extra blood churning through the system is likely to keep you awake. In fact, if you're heading out on the town, one of the best things to eat to pick up your pace is dark chocolate–covered cocoa nibs (available at www.TheChocolateTherapist.com/buycacao.php).

Chamomile tea is recommended with the "slightly" dark chocolate (55%) because this tea has been used as a calming aid for centuries. The lower level of dark chocolate will also provide less theobromine. The two together should bring about a calming lineup of semisweet dreams.

Additional considerations: no yelling at anyone after 2:00 P.M. (no exceptions here), no vigorous exercise after 8:00 P.M., and no plate throwing at any time; more candles and instrumental music in the evening and one weekly dinner out with your significant other to avoid the potentially aggravating (and thus heart-racing) discussion of who will do the dishes.

Lack of Sexual Desire

Recommendation

Share 1 entire bar of dark chocolate with almonds with your partner in bed while reading poetry by candlelight. Optional activities may be indulged in when you have finished medicating.

Supporting Evidence

Not surprisingly, the research for arousing sexual desire is almost the same as that found in the "Heartbreak" section. Unfortunately, the two often go hand in hand. As previously mentioned, chocolate contains small amounts of a nervous system stimulant called phenylethylamine. PEA is the chemical the body releases when people experience the rush of falling in love, and a substantial increase of PEA occurs in the brain during orgasm. PEA also helps trigger neurotransmitters in the brain that make us happy—in fact, studies have shown that happy people have considerably more PEA in their brains than do those who are unhappy. Adding a little chocolate to your relationship mix is bound to produce some stimulating effects!

Here's an interesting study from the *Journal of Sexual Medicine*. To discover whether daily chocolate consumption increased sexual desire, a group of researchers asked 163 Italian women questions about chocolate consumption and desire. After consolidating the results, researchers concluded that women who ate more chocolate did experience more desire, but chocolate consumption was also directly related to age: younger women ate more chocolate and also reported more desire.

Of course, the researchers stated that age directly correlates to sexual desire, but the inquiring mind could take the concept a bit further. Did the older women lose their desire because they cut back on chocolate? Did they cut back on chocolate to lose weight? Did they gain weight because they cut back on sex? And why weren't men included in the study?

Regarding the men, my theory is that no company would consider funding research to determine whether young men have sexual desire, regardless of their chocolate consumption. We may never know the actual answer to the other questions. Why take a risk? Just eat your dark chocolate and see what happens. Indulge in the recommended bar, and you'll benefit from the almonds as well. One study maintained that eating 10–20 almonds a day invigorates sexual desire.

If you're really in a quandary, eat a tablespoon of raw organic cacao nibs (www.TheChocolateTherapist.com/buycacao.php) about an hour before your rendezvous. After all, Montezuma didn't drink a reported fifty cups of cocoa a day before attending to his harem *only* because he liked the taste.

Lactose Intolerance

Recommendation

Take 3 squares dairy-free dark chocolate whenever the mood strikes, up to a maximum of 9 squares per day.

Supporting Evidence

If you love milk but your body doesn't, this could be the answer for you. Researchers from the University of Rhode Island demonstrated that adding 1½ teaspoons of cocoa to milk reduced and sometimes even eliminated cramping and bloating in half of their lactose-intolerant subjects. It appears that chocolate stimulates the enzyme lactase, which is required for lactose digestion.

Most dark chocolate is lactose-free, anyway. This is where reading labels comes in handy once again. A few popular mainstream brands actually put milk fat in their dark chocolate, but a simple review of the wrapper can resolve the potential dilemma. The recommendation still calls for dairy-free chocolate to ensure that you don't aggravate the condition. If you find you've inadvertently ingested something that contains lactose or milk, however, consider using dark chocolate to help ease your symptoms.

Life Expectancy

Recommendation

One dark chocolate bar (organic is ideal) of your choice, daily, for the rest of your life. Keep alcohol to a minimum, don't smoke, drive safely, relax, and drink plenty of pure spring water.

Supporting Evidence

Thank you, Harvard, for supplying the chocolate lovers of the world with this invaluable information. After studying 7,841 male graduates for eighteen years, the Harvard School of Public Health reported that people who eat chocolate live nearly a year longer than do those who attempt to go through life without the luxury.

My theory is that chocolate lovers intentionally hang on for an extra year so that they can enjoy chocolate for another 365 days! This could quite possibly be the single most important reason to make sure there's adequate chocolate in your diet. You'll average an extra year to enjoy the fruits of the cocoa bean in its many varied splendors, as well as anything else you like to do.

If one additional year isn't long enough, add nuts to your daily chocolate dose. Research conducted at the Public School of Health at Loma Linda University concluded that adding nuts to the diet is one of the variables associated with longevity. It works out nicely, because nuts are chocolate's perfect partner when pairing.

Macular Degeneration

Recommendation

Take 3–4 tablespoons raw dark chocolate–covered cocoa nibs daily with 10 walnuts and a steaming cup of antioxidant tea any time before noon.

Supporting Evidence

This unfortunate disease generally strikes people over fifty. It's characterized by a gradual loss of sight in the macula, or the center of the eye. Reading and recognition of others become increasingly difficult.

Nearly all degenerative disease is caused in some way by free radicals—destructive molecules that float around in the bloodstream and attack healthy cells. Macular degeneration is particularly affected by this type of destruction, and an antioxidant-rich diet can be very helpful in combating the effects. As I've mentioned many times, chocolate contains some of the highest levels of antioxidants by weight of all foods. In fact, chocolate has been listed as one of the top "superfoods" in numerous nutritional publications.

The rate of macular degeneration also rises among people who have a higher intake of unhealthy fats. Conversely, when people eat more healthy fats—particularly, omega-3 essential fatty acids—the incidence of macular degeneration is lower.

Most people know that fish oil and flaxseed oil are two of the highest sources of omega-3, but these two items don't taste particularly delicious with chocolate, at least not in their fishy and oily forms. A quick review of omega 3–rich nuts and foods yielded the following preferable options for pairing with chocolate: flaxseeds, English walnuts, and black walnuts, in that order.

Overall, I found the advice on preventing macular degeneration a bit limited—plenty of information but not too many conclusive statistics. Yet keep in mind that when the body breaks down and begins to function improperly, the root cause lies in its inability to generate fully functioning cells. Over time, broken cells create broken bodies. Omega-3 fats have been shown time and again to help cells regenerate properly. A light snack of chocolate, walnuts, and antioxidant-rich tea will certainly help the cells in general, and if they're misbehaving in the vision area, it's likely to help there as well.

Memory Loss

Recommendation

Take 4 squares dark chocolate with optional pine nuts and sunflower seeds as a midmorning snack and again in between lunch and dinner. May be consumed with tea, water, or hot chocolate (see the recipe in chapter 9).

Supporting Evidence

Memory experts have shown that eating a little of the right kind of chocolate each day can actually help improve your memory. Dark chocolate contains an antioxidant called procyanidin that helps block the effect of two aging factors in the brain: oxidation and inflammation. These same procyanidins may also help memory by stimulating circulation in the brain. Increased blood flow delivers more oxygen and nutrients to the brain, helping to maintain optimal functioning.

Chocolate contains a number of vitamins that are known to benefit the brain, particularly vitamin B1 (thiamin). Thiamin helps produce energy and maintain proper psychological functioning. A *British Journal of Psychiatry* study showed that as many of 30 percent of people entering mental institutions were deficient in thiamin. Another report in the *Journal of Geriatric Psychology and Neurology* showed improved mental performance in Alzheimer's patients who were given therapeutic levels of thiamin (3–8 grams) daily.

Once again, a quick reminder that to get *any* benefit at all from chocolate, you must consume dark chocolate because all of the benefits are in the cocoa powder. The amount of vitamins is relatively small. To put things into perspective, a person would have to consume 5.47 pounds of chocolate a day to meet the U.S. Recommended Daily Allowance of 1.5 grams of thiamine. Obviously, this is slightly more per day than would be considered health-promoting—in fact, more than 5 pounds over the limit.

The purpose of running the numbers is to help you remember that most studies subject participants to therapeutic doses and subsequently report generic cross data that lead you to believe that eating this *one* food can produce miracles for you. Everything you eat contributes to your well-being. It's the combination of high-quality, nutrient-rich whole foods eaten at every meal that creates health—not focusing on *one* product because you saw a study or two that supports what you want to eat.

The moral of the story: when eating chocolate, always choose dark chocolate that contains 60% or more cocoa. Health-wise consumers will also eat chocolate with nuts, spices, dried fruits, and organic flavoring oils in lieu of those with sugary centers, preservatives, and artificial flavors.

Menopause

Recommendation

Call an older friend or two, snap off half a 75% dark chocolate bar with nuts and dried fruit (optional but good for a lift), pour a glass of Australian Shiraz, and clear the area of men for 30 minutes to 1 hour of girl-talk therapy.

Supporting Evidence

Studies show that many women crave chocolate once menopause sets in. After reading through the statistics, you'll have no guilt about heading to the kitchen for your hormone balancer (even if you're premenopausal, I suspect). Seventy percent of us will have at least some kind of symptoms, so it's better to learn to manage them than spend time hoping you'll be on the good side of the statistic. I once heard a quote that seems appropriate: "Hope is not a strategy."

Menopause is caused by the age-related reduction of two hormones: estrogen and progesterone. Younger bodies produce adequate amounts for ovulation, but as we age we produce less. Over time, the end result is menopause, or the ceasing of regular menstruation. Although there is some obvious relief to be gained, plenty of new troublesome issues arrive, such as night sweats, hot flashes, raging mood swings, a higher risk for heart problems, and many more.

Enter chocolate. As mentioned later in the "PMS" section, chocolate contains naturally high levels of magnesium, which help regulate hormones—particularly progesterone. A single bar supplies as much as 15 percent of your daily magnesium requirement. Considering that the majority of all women are magnesium-deficient, there's a good reason that you're craving chocolate. It contains many of the same benefits for menopause that it does for PMS.

Just like all of the recommendations, it's important to eat high-quality dark chocolate to get all of the benefits. A report from the *Journal of Cardiovascular Pharmacology* demonstrated that postmenopausal women who were given flavanol-rich chocolate (high in antioxidants) had improved vascular function, while those who had low-flavanol chocolate (poor-quality chocolate, low in antioxidants) didn't experience any positive results at all. Choose chocolate with cocoa butter instead of milk fat, butter fat, or vegetable oil, and you'll get healthy fats instead of cholesterol-raising fats.

Adding nuts to your chocolate can be helpful as well, because nuts contain vitamin E, a long-time natural remedy for women suffering from hot flashes. Yet not everyone agrees on this strategy. On its Web site, the Mayo Clinic states that vitamin E is no longer recommended for hot flashes. But a report in *Gynecologic and Obstetric Investigation* (*GOI*) disagrees, saying that as little as 400 IU per day can reduce hot flashes.

Controversy runs deep from one report to the next, and in all of this fuss, I discovered an interesting research blunder. The *GOI* research that supports the use of vitamin E for menopause actually references research from the Mayo Clinic to substantiate its findings, making one wonder just exactly where the Mayo Clinic stands on the subject. A slightly altered phrase from the beloved Shakespeare comes to mind: To E or not to E—*that* is the question.

In general, the Mayo Clinic recommended lifestyle and diet changes, yet disregarded traditional remedies such as black cohosh, soy, red clover, and vitamin supplements. The Mayo Clinic authors endorsed newer medications that have offered relief to sufferers, such as antidepressants, the seizure medicine Gabapentin, and the high blood pressure medicine Clonidine. Of course, there are just as many reports to support natural remedies, but no one is paying big dollars to have popular health-focused Web sites endorse them, which is why we see more and more recommendations for drug use and fewer for natural supplements.

The results of taking vitamin E for menopause undoubtedly differ based on the quantity consumed, as well as on the type used (natural d-alpha-tocopherol is the only form the body can absorb), but not surprisingly, many of the reports fail to mention these crucial details. Why? I suspect the same reason as mentioned previously: the studies are paid for by companies that want you to use hormone-replacement therapy or drugs.

Ultimately, the best study for you is the one you do on yourself—try taking 400–800 IU of vitamin E (only d-alpha will do, not dl-alpha) and eat vitamin E–rich foods for ninety days and see what happens. You have peace of life to gain and nothing to lose, except hot flashes, of course.

Mental Performance

Recommendation

Take ½ 60%+ dark chocolate bar with acai and blueberries 30–60 minutes prior to performing tasks that require mental acuity. Optional: drink 8 ounces hot chocolate made using the recipe in chapter 9.

Supporting Evidence

Schoolteachers take note! Researchers at the University of Nottingham in England discovered that flavanol-rich drinks increased blood flow to the brain, providing more oxygen and nutrients and raising overall mental performance. The effects lasted for two to three hours, suggesting that if you're going to gain any benefit from chocolate for mental performance, you'd best perform your mental tasks within that time period. Note: a large chocolate bar eaten the night before a test will most likely not help.

Another interesting study from Wheeling Jesuit University in West Virginia found that subjects who consumed 85 grams of chocolate (both dark and milk were tested) fifteen minutes prior to cognitive testing performed up to 20 percent better than the unlucky half of participants who were not given chocolate. Performance evaluations were made on word discrimination, verbal memory, design memory, attention span, reaction time, problem solving, and response variability. Overall, the study showed "improved impulse control and reaction time," with milk chocolate results higher than dark.

I do not, however, recommend milk chocolate because it has too much sugar and fat. If you plan to eat chocolate to improve mental performance, eat dark chocolate for the best overall results. Also, 85 grams of chocolate in a single setting is significantly more than one should eat daily for health, so keep the chocolate consumption used in this study limited to big test emergencies, such as medical exams, law school admission tests, finals, and checkers with grandma.

Older people demonstrated cognitive benefits from chocolate consumption as well. A study conducted by the Department of

Nutrition in Oslo, Norway, compared the effects of chocolate, tea, and red wine consumption on cognitive performance on 2,031 subjects between the ages of 70 and 74. When given a variety of tests, those who consumed all three food items had the highest test scores. The wine drinkers were actually the highest, with chocolate and tea drinkers coming in slightly lower. The object of the test was to determine whether flavonoid-rich foods positively affected cognitive performance, and the results showed that they did.

Mood Swings

Recommendation

Take 6 squares dark organic chocolate with or without nuts at the onset of any bad mood. It's acceptable to count picking up kids' clothes and an overstuffed garage as possible attitude triggers.

Supporting Evidence

Like the remedy for "Sassy Kids" (see later), chocolate offers the ultimate one-two punch with its physiological and emotional benefits. In his book *Naked Chocolate*, chocolate enthusiast David Wolfe gives an extraordinarily comprehensive summary of the properties of chocolate. Natural chemicals that positively affect moods include phenylethylamine, anandamide, and tryptophan. Chocolate also helps the body release serotonin, the primary neurotransmitter for mood stability, and dopamine, another neurotransmitter that enhances mood and promotes relaxation. In addition to all of these psychological boosters, the fat content of chocolate satiates the appetite, and its flavor compounds satisfy a diverse assortment of cravings.

Chocolate also has a number of positive emotional connections. Love and chocolate often arrive in the same bite, thanks to chocolate's association with Valentine's Day. In fact, many people associate good feelings with eating chocolate and occasionally even with the mere sight of it. Chocolate melts perfectly at body temperature. Once it's in the mouth, the smooth, creamy texture feels soft, warm, and delicious, obviously initiating more feel-good sensations.

The delightful mélange of benefits in chocolate makes it the ultimate mood-manipulating snack. But be aware that an innocent indulgence can easily explode into its own drastic mood swing without a bit of discipline. As the cliché so appropriately states, Too much of a good thing is a bad thing.

To avoid a possible overindulgence, keep consumption limited to the recommended amounts and especially eat *dark* chocolate instead of milk chocolate to keep your blood sugar level low. Too much sugar can make your moods worse. Once you've hit the six-square limit, try a series of other mood busters, such as drinking 16 ounces of water, taking a B-complex vitamin, doing some deep-breathing exercises, watching a funny movie, or eating a bowl of organic baby carrots with ranch dressing (no research on that last one . . . just an idea).

Optional: if you're truly in a tirade, consider staying away from loved ones to avoid making necessary apologies later.

Nausea / Speaking in Public

Recommendation

Take ½ bar dark chocolate with mint with 1 cup mint tea. Use peppermint mints shortly before speaking engagements. Look into the mirror prior to stepping on the podium to ensure that you have a chocolate-free face to reduce the possibility of embarrassment.

Supporting Evidence

Not only does chocolate contain the calming amino acid tryptophan, but it also stimulates the release of serotonin and dopamine into the brain, two neurotransmitters that promote relaxation. Because a relaxed state of mind is ideal for public speaking, a good-quality dark chocolate bar can be very helpful. Add nuts and it doubles as a healthy snack, which is good for speakers who can't or choose not to eat a full meal before lecturing.

Adding mint to your chocolate offers additional relief because it has been used for centuries as a digestive aid. Mint has a unique ability to calm the body's smooth muscles, allowing it to benefit a number of areas where digestive aggravation is a problem. According to World's Healthiest Foods (www.WHFoods.com), peppermint's healing properties include alleviating colonic muscle spasms, irritable bowel syndrome, indigestion, and dyspepsia. It has also been used to lessen morning sickness, menstrual cramps, and nausea, including the type induced by public-speaking engagements.

Even after a night of heavy drinking, try this prescription for measurable relief to calm the stomach. Herbal Hangover Cure (www.LifeScript.com) notes that mint leaves can either be chewed or brewed to help calm a queasy stomach. But for maximum benefit, stick with the recommendation of both tea *and* chocolate. You'll need the extra antioxidant punch of the chocolate to help neutralize the deluge of alcohol-induced free radicals that helped cause the nausea in the first place.

Osteoporosis

Recommendation

Take 4 squares milk chocolate (with or without almonds) and 1 cup hot cocoa (see the recipe in chapter 9) midmorning 4–5 days per week.

Supporting Evidence

Chocolate contains both calcium and magnesium—two minerals that are deficient in many people's diets. Women in particular do not meet the U.S. Recommended Daily Allowance for trace elements. Of course, you can't prevent osteoporosis by consuming immense quantities of chocolate. Yet by following the recommendation exactly, the odds of becoming calcium-deficient can be moved in your favor. The cup of milk provides 30 percent of your daily calcium requirement, and the magnesium in chocolate helps the body with calcium absorption.

Recent research suggests that adding dairy products to chocolate decreases the body's ability to make use of its antioxidants. To ensure that you obtain both antioxidant and calcium benefits from chocolate, you may want to consider substituting rice or soy milk for regular milk. Both of these products also contain an estimated 30 percent of the daily requirement for calcium.

There are two chocolate options in the recommendation—one with and one without almonds. Almonds provide an excellent collection of minerals associated with building bone density—calcium, magnesium, manganese, and phosphorous. Regardless of which bar you choose, eat it with the prescribed chocolate milk of your choice for maximum benefits.

PMS

Recommendation

On days 14–25 of your cycle, take ¼ (2 ounces) high-quality dark chocolate bar daily after lunch or whenever food cravings hit, limiting your intake to ½ bar per day. On days 25–28, consume up to an entire bar per day, as needed, to curb cravings, crabbiness, and lethargy.

Supporting Evidence

Studies have shown that many women use chocolate to self-medicate during this often stressful time of the month. This is hardly breaking news. I don't know of a woman who *doesn't* use chocolate during this time of the month. There's no need to examine the reasons we use it. A simple review of many of the other ailments in this book will address the issue. After all, it appears that PMS is a compilation of every conceivable symptom packed into a three- to five-day slice of the month.

One physical cause of PMS is a drop in the hormone progesterone, a change that can bring about nasty mood swings, hot flashes, and a host of other miserable symptoms. Adding magnesium to the diets of women affected with chronic PMS symptoms helps alleviate the problem by increasing premenstrual progesterone levels. Because chocolate has one of the highest concentrations of natural magnesium, it makes sense that we would naturally crave it during this time of the month. It contains the very thing to help stabilize our fluctuating hormones.

Serotonin also drops during the course of the month. It maintains a fairly normal level until approximately day 14, when it begins a steady downward path. By the last few days of the cycle, serotonin levels are at their lowest. This creates a more pronounced desire for something like chocolate that will lift your mood. Conveniently, chocolate contains substances that stimulate the body to release serotonin into the system.

In addition, levels of endorphins in your body zoom up and down the chart during the month. They actually spike within forty-eight hours of ovulation, drifting back down to a normal level toward the end of the cycle. The disheartening synopsis: not only does the body experience a drop in progesterone and serotonin by month's end, but it also suffers from the withdrawal of endorphin euphoria. Fortunately, eating chocolate triggers the release of endorphins in the body, which can help ease this plunge.

Because chocolate helps curb both the mental and the physiological symptoms of PMS, be prepared! This is your opportunity to get the best chocolate collection from your sweetie. A well-placed list of your favorite chocolate bars (i.e., on the refrigerator door or taped to a six-pack) just prior to that "special" time of the month will give him plenty of opportunity to prepare. If you're lacking a significant other, permission is granted to treat yourself. Have plenty of high-quality dark chocolate on hand. It's better to snap off the corner of a chocolate bar than your significant other's head.

Also make a note to avoid caffeine, sugary treats, fried foods, and alcohol. Starchy processed foods have a tendency to trigger a rise in estrogen, making it too high relative to progesterone—another cause of PMS.

Pregnancy

Recommendation

Take 4 squares dark chocolate daily while massaging cocoa butter onto the abdominal area to help prevent stretch marks.

Supporting Evidence

Let's face it: there isn't much that will stave off the snarling moods of a challenging pregnancy, and it's safe to say that many pregnancies are just that. It would be nice to think that chocolate could get the job done, but short of having the baby, there's only one thing you can do while the time passes: endure.

This is where chocolate comes in because, after all, nearly everything is a little more bearable when chocolate is involved. Fortunately, most doctors don't advise against eating chocolate while pregnant, although there's still that nasty little rumor that it contains too much caffeine. But recall from "Caffeine Withdrawal" that chocolate has virtually no caffeine—much less in a single bar than in a cup of decaf. Instead, it contains theobromine, another central nervous system stimulant with a milder effect on the body.

One interesting study showed that women who consumed chocolate during pregnancy had an inversely related incidence of preeclampsia. In layman's terms, that means, "The more chocolate they ate, the lower the incidence of preeclampsia." But don't misinterpret the statistic to mean that you have permission to undertake a carte-blanche chocolate eating plan for nine solid months. Moderation is always essential.

What about the baby and chocolate? Researchers in Finland followed 305 women during their pregnancies, some of whom ate chocolate and others who didn't. Subjects who enjoyed a little chocolate every day reported having happier babies at six months than those who didn't eat chocolate. In this case, chocolate consumption was definitely a double-positive: eat chocolate and have a happy baby or don't eat chocolate and baby is not as happy.

Overall, "chocolate" and "pregnancy" fit safely in the same sentence. Most of the research supports moderate indulgence while pregnant. But that could be said of everything from steak tartar to double-dark peanut butter chocolate ice cream, to fried green tomatoes, all of which you may be inspired to enjoy during this fabulous chapter of your life.

Prostate Cancer

Recommendation

Men should take 5 chocolate-covered coffee beans daily after age forty, which is when prostate cancer begins to be a statistically significant risk.

Supporting Evidence

According to a study reported in the *European Journal of Cancer Prevention*, a compound derived from chocolate polyphenol extracts called Acticoa powder effectively protected rats from prostate carcinogens when given "chronically" before the test. Note that "chronically" means given daily or consistently. If you eat chocolate on Sundays, you'll benefit only on Sunday. Eat it on holidays, you'll benefit on holidays. As chocolate studies often use "chronic" consumption for their results, do the same to get the same results.

It's also interesting to note that the rats were given the Acticoa powder for two weeks before the test. Those that fared best had consumed a moderate amount of the powder, compared to those that were given larger amounts or none at all. Moderation is another key to success.

Coffee beans are recommended because of research supporting an inverse relationship between coffee consumption and cancer. Specifically, the Channing Laboratory/Harvard Medical School study followed fifty thousand men for twenty years, concluding that those who drank the most coffee had a significantly lower incidence of lethal prostate cancer. In an unrelated study, tall men will also be relieved to discover that a study to determine whether height increased prostate cancer risk concluded that the relationship was insignificant. How do researchers come up with these ideas? What about short men, bald men, nice men, rich men, pilots, scientists, or pastors?

Sassy Kids

Recommendation

Give the child ½ bar high-quality dark or milk chocolate, with or without nuts, as needed, preferably after meals or as a reward for improved behavior.

Supporting Evidence

Controlling children by manipulating them with chocolate treats may seem like a questionable idea at first glance. Yet many people already use food-based rewards to encourage good behavior. The issue is more about the *type* of food given, not whether to give food as a reward.

Kids usually act out when they're tired, hungry, or in a bad mood. It's easy to buy the nearest treat in sight to get some peace. Children seem to know this because they gravitate toward quick fixes filled with dyes, white sugar, and preservatives. But if you're going to let them have a treat, consider making it good-quality chocolate instead of the first box of candy you see.

Chocolate offers an excellent one-two remedy for sassy kids. The tryptophan in chocolate encourages the release of serotonin, a neurotransmitter that creates calmness and mood stability. Fat stimulates the release of endorphins, natural brain chemicals that promote energy and euphoria. The fat also enters the bloodstream much more slowly than the pure-sugar treats, which helps keep blood sugar stable and prevents the post–sugar crash yo-yo syndrome.

Add this to all of the other benefits that children get from chocolate—antioxidants, a few vitamins, minerals, and a host of flavor compounds—and you've just solved a problem with a healthy treat. Of course, kids may get the picture and act out more often in an attempt to receive more chocolate. To overcome this possible hazard, simply give them a few squares every day to regulate mood swings and promote euphoria (for the children, as well as for the parents).

Note: milk chocolate is recommended for kids because they seem to prefer its milder flavor; however, don't hesitate to help the little darlings switch over to dark chocolate as soon as possible. The sooner they learn to enjoy dark chocolate, the better for everyone. Also, milk chocolate should not be consumed daily because it contains too much sugar. Milk chocolate is good for an occasional treat, but the daily plan should feature dark chocolate.

Smoking Cessation

Recommendation

Take 1½ ounces extremely dark chocolate (75%+) with an optional 2-ounce shot of guava juice daily until you kick the habit, after which you can reduce your intake to 1¼ ounces per day. People attempting to quit smoking can improve their willpower and success rate by adding 6 or more 8-ounce glasses of pure water to their daily intake.

Supporting Evidence

The *Journal of the American College of Cardiology* recently reported that the consumption of chocolate may reverse some of the artery damage caused by smoking. Nicotine constricts blood vessels, adversely affecting blood's ability to flow smoothly. Over time, nicotine abuse can cause thrombosis and atherosclerosis, among many other health problems. Compounds in chocolate encourage the body to release nitric oxide into the blood, which helps dilate blood vessels. Similar benefits are reviewed in the "High Blood Pressure" and "Heart Disease" sections.

Numerous studies have shown that the smoke from only one cigarette bombards the body with millions of free radicals, causing serious damage on many levels. The body's own natural defense system can't even begin to combat the assault. It needs extra help, and eating antioxidant-rich foods is one of the best solutions. The abundant antioxidants in chocolate scavenge excess free radicals from the body and protect it from the many harmful side effects of smoking. Antioxidants work double duty because they also help repair tissue damage caused by smoking.

The *Harvard Men's Health Watch* recently devoted an entire section to chocolate and how it benefits health, including recent research conducted in Germany about chocolate and smoking. Researchers discovered that flavanol-rich cocoa actually helps reverse some of the endothelial (inner artery lining) damage caused by smoking. The report also cited research showing how dark chocolate helped reduce blood pressure and blood clotting and improved insulin sensitivity.

The optional shot of guava juice is recommended for its high content of vitamin C, a potent antioxidant that has been shown to prevent oxidation of LDLs. LDL oxidation is one of the primary causes of atherosclerosis, a disease often present in smokers. Vitamin C also helps regenerate vitamin E in the body, which is another powerful antioxidant that can help overcome the massive free radical deluge the body experiences from cigarettes.

People who are really committed to quitting should add the recommended amount of water to their daily regimen, as suggested earlier. In his top-selling diet book *Get with the Program*, author Bob Greene lists many reasons hydration can help smokers get their nicotine habit under control.

Sniffles

Recommendation

Take 3–6 squares dark chocolate with mint daily just after a chicken soup lunch until symptoms subside. Do not exceed a maximum of 12 squares in a 24-hour period.

Supporting Evidence

Colds need plenty of pampering, and chocolate with mint is just the "mother" you need. The antioxidants in chocolate help your immune system combat colds. Adding mint to your chocolate is beneficial because peppermint relaxes the breathing passages.

Peppermint is used in many teas to combat nasal congestion, stuffiness, hay fever, sinusitis, and allergies by helping to restore breathing.

Your mother may have rubbed Vicks VapoRub on your chest when you had a cold as a child, but the updated technique is eating chocolate with mint (not smearing it on your chest, of course, although that's optional). If you enjoy it with the recommended mint tea, you'll get the added benefit of having a warm mouth to melt the chocolate and accentuate the flavors.

Spousal Discord

Recommendation

Enjoy Chocolate Kahlua Truffles by candlelight with soft music and a glass of red wine with your significant other (see the recipe in chapter 9). Children in the area will most likely counteract the effects, so it's best to do this in a dimly lit, private location.

Supporting Evidence

Chocolate, love, passion, and romance. The four clearly go hand in hand, a concept that obviously doesn't need scientific proof to back it up. If you need to spice up your spouse, consider the following: chocolate stimulates the flow of feel-good chemicals in the brain, and it contains the same natural substance (PEA) that the brain releases when you fall in love. It also contains tryptophan, an amino acid that promotes relaxation. In addition, tryptophan is the precursor to the body's primary neurotransmitter serotonin, which calms the body and staves off anxiety. With its sensual characteristic of melting at body temperature and its vast array of rich, complex, velvety flavors, chocolate *is* passion. Here are a few recommendations to help you reconnect with your loved one:

If you need to say:

"I love you": A bar of high-grade dark chocolate and a red rose laid across the top.

"I'm sorry": A larger bar of high-quality dark organic chocolate and a thoughtful apology on a handmade card.

"Let's have fun": An exotically flavored large dark chocolate bar that can be broken into individual squares and fed to your partner, as needed, while playing games of intimacy. Sensual scented candles are optional.

"You are the best person in the world!": Decorate your significant other's office (or favorite room) with various types of chocolate wrapped in colorful paper. Place a copy of *The Chocolate Therapist*, tied with a tastefully selected ribbon, on the center of your sweetie's desk. Follow your intuition.

Stress

Recommendation

Take ½ bar dark chocolate with vanilla essence directly after lunch every Monday, when stress is likely to be at a high point. Repeat as needed during the week, but always on Mondays.

Supporting Evidence

Chocolate contains potassium and magnesium, as well as several vitamins such as B1, B2, D, and E. Magnesium, the hero nutrient in chocolate, helps regulate the pituitary gland and keep the adrenal glands in check. When the adrenals function properly, you're much more able to handle the daily stressors of life. B vitamins also become depleted in the body under stressful situations. Eating a good-quality chocolate bar can help replenish a few of the nutrients you lose due to stress.

In addition, chocolate stimulates the release of endorphins, natural chemicals in the brain that promote calm and euphoric feelings. There's even a substance in chocolate called anandamide, which affects the same areas of the brain that marijuana does. Anandamide actually stays in the brain longer, prolonging the relaxed sensation in a completely safe and natural way. The amount of anandamide in chocolate is very small, but it's measurable in the brain after chocolate consumption. Still, there's no need for concern—a person would have to eat twenty-five pounds of chocolate to feel the same "high" that would occur from smoking one joint. Fortunately, it looks as if chocolate will remain a legal substance for many years to come.

A number of brands offer chocolate selections with vanilla essence, which is recommended because of the calming benefits of vanilla. This scent is used in aromatherapy to relax the body. For the true chocolate adventurer, carrot juice has proved to be particularly effective in helping to relieve stress as well. For a high-powered meeting, consider serving organic baby carrots dipped in melted dark chocolate instead of doughnuts. It may not help you close the deal, but it will certainly make for some interesting conversation. On second thought, it may help close the deal as well.

Stroke

Recommendation

Take 1 ounce dark chocolate with 1 tablespoon each dried orange peel bits and hemp seeds. The seeds and the orange peel can either be eaten separately or melted into the chocolate.

Supporting Evidence

Before anyone panics when reading this recommendation, there are no psychoactive elements in hemp seeds, unlike those that come to mind when we think of other hemp-related products. Hemp seeds are legal and can be purchased in most natural grocery stores. By weight, they're also one of the most protein-rich and essential fatty acid (EFA) balanced seeds available. They're included in the recommendation because consuming EFAs has been shown to be inversely related to the incidence of stroke.

A stroke is caused by a cessation of blood flow to critical areas of the brain, disrupting functioning and often resulting in temporary or permanent disability. According to the American Stroke Association, strokes are the third leading cause of death in the United States (behind heart disease and cancer), they occur every forty seconds, and they happen more often to women than to men.

People with high cholesterol and/or high blood pressure are statistically at a higher risk of having a stroke than those with normal levels. There is significant research about chocolate and blood-pressure reduction, as reviewed in "High Blood Pressure." Because dark chocolate helps with both of these conditions, it benefits the body by lessening the incidence of stroke as well.

Orange peel is recommended because of its high content of vitamin C, a vitamin that has been shown to reduce the likelihood of suffering a stroke. In a study reported in the *American Journal of Clinical Nutrition*, researchers studied more than 20,000 people for over nine years. Of this group, 448 people had strokes during the study. On evaluation, researchers discovered that those who had the highest blood levels of vitamin C had a 42 percent lower risk of having a stroke. Inversely, subjects who had the lowest blood levels of vitamin C had the greatest incidence of strokes.

To maximize your risk reduction for strokes, move to Colorado, New Mexico, or Arizona. According to the latest (2006) demographics map that's available from the American Stroke Association, these three states have the lowest stroke-related death rates in the nation.

(Interestingly enough, Colorado is the only state that comes in lowest in cardiovascular disease, heart disease, and stroke. As a longtime resident myself, I can see that most of us embrace very healthy lifestyles. So, are we healthier because we live here, or do we choose to live here because we're healthy? This is an ideal time to find out which comes first, and, of course, the best way is to move here and do your own research. You'll be forced to enjoy 320 days of sun per year, play outside with us, and work less. I know it's a commitment, but someone has to do it.)

Sugar Overload

Recommendation

Take ½ bar of the strongest dark chocolate you can tolerate, preferably 70%+ cocoa. Divide the bar into sections, and enjoy a few throughout the day. Add 500 milligrams of the amino acid l-glutamine daily to help curb sugar cravings.

Supporting Evidence

According to an article published at www.HealingDaily.com, the average American consumes 135 pounds of sugar per year. That's a conservative estimate, according to a recent release of *Get the Sugar Out*, by Ann Louise Gittleman, which states that the average annual consumption is up to 180 pounds. Another source, www.Diet-plans.org, reported that the average daily sugar intake for male U.S. teens is 34 teaspoons per day. An Australian site reported that Aussies consume approximately 31 teaspoons a day, and a Malaysian site sent an alarming message to its citizens that diabetes had increased 400 percent within just the last five years.

These are only a few of the many countries concerned about their increasing sugar consumption and the subsequent surge in disease.

One reason sugar intake is on the rise is that stress is on the rise. We're looking for quick fixes to increase our feeling of well-being. Sugar is the easy answer because it helps the brain release serotonin—our primary feel-good neurotransmitter that keeps stress at bay. Unfortunately, sugar causes far more harm than good in the body. Sugar even has similar characteristics to other addictive substances, such as a need to consume more over time to achieve the same "feel-good" effects.

When the bills add up, the kids are fighting, the market tumbles, and the world economy crashes, something sweet often seems like it's the only answer! The best strategy is to find a food that satisfies the need for a treat without adding to your daily sugar overload.

Enter dark chocolate. True, it's somewhat counterintuitive. If you're trying to avoid or cut down on sugar, it stands to reason that a new plan of eating *more* chocolate will never work. Yet a good-quality dark chocolate bar doesn't contain nearly as much sugar as some of the other, more "acceptable" snacks. After comparing the grams of sugar in the listed foods, you may want to reconsider allowing chocolate back into the snack cupboard.

Food	Grams of Sugar per Serving
Extra dark chocolate bar	12 (varies slightly depending on brand)
⅓ cup Craisins	26
1 cup Life cereal	12
16 ounces Gatorade	26
Nature Valley Chewy Granola Bar	13
1 can Coca-Cola	27
1 small Hershey's brownie	17
1 Yoplait fat-free yogurt	15

It's difficult to completely eliminate sugar from the diet, especially when you're beginning a new diet and attempting to go cold turkey. According to Holly McCord, a nutritionist and the author of *Win the Sugar War*, moderation is superior to elimination and much more realistic. It's been proved that as soon as you try to remove anything from your diet, you're likely to start craving it more than ever. Better to take on a reduction plan and move toward a lower intake level over time. When you're starting a new diet, try eating a little very dark chocolate to avert cravings or binges triggered by sugar withdrawal (see "Food Cravings" for additional information).

What about sugar-free foods? Many companies offer chocolates made with sugar-free sweeteners, but don't go overboard just because they're sugar-free. Eating too many of these bars in one sitting will have you referring to the "Flatulence" section. The ingredient that is used to replace sugar (usually, maltitol) tends to cause indigestion and gas. Many sugar-free chocolates also contain sweeteners such as aspartame and saccharin, which are known toxins to the body. It's much healthier to eat good-quality, high–cocoa content chocolate than sugar-free chocolate.

Vitamin Deficiency

Recommendation

Take 3 squares dark chocolate with breakfast 3 days per week, along with your daily morning vitamins.

Supporting Evidence

The following chart shows the nutritional content of a dark chocolate bar. I compared the fat and calorie values for the listed bar to the chocolate recommended throughout the book, and it's clear that the bar used for this information is inferior to high-quality dark chocolate. The researchers didn't specify the exact type of chocolate they used, but had it been a higher-quality dark chocolate bar, the results of this chart would be even higher in nutrients.

Nutrients in Dark Chocolate			
Nutrient	Unit	Value/ 100 g	1 Bar/ 44 g
Energy	Kcal	479	210.76
Protein	G	4.20	1.85
Total lipid (fat)	G	30	13.20
Carbohydrate	G	63.10	27.76
Fiber, dietary	G	5.9	2.60
Sugars, total	G	54.50	23.98
Calcium	Mg	32.00	14.08
Iron	Mg	3.13	1.38
Magnesium	Mg	115.00	50.60
Phosphorus	Mg	1132.00	58.08
Potassium	Mg	365.00	160.60
Sodium	Mg	11.00	4.84
Zinc	Mg	1.62	0.71
Copper	Mg	0.70	0.31
Manganese	Mg	.80	0.35
Selenium	Mcg	3.10	1.36
Vitamin C	Mg	0.00	0.00
Thiamin	Mg	0.06	0.02
Riboflavin	Mg	0.09	0.04
Niacin	Mg	0.43	0.19
Pantothenic acid	Mg	0.11	0.05

Vitamin B6	Mg	0.034	0.02
Vitamin A, IU	IU	21.00	9.24
Vitamin A, RE	Mcg_RE	2.00	0.88
Vitamin E	Mg_ATE	1.19	0.52
Fatty acids, saturated	G	17.75	7.81
Fatty acids, unsaturated	G	0.97	0.43
Cholesterol	Mg	0	0
Caffeine	Mg	62.00	22.28
Theobromine	Mg	486.00	213.84

From the USDA Nutrient Database for Standard Reference, Release 13 (November 1999).

Two of the most abundant and beneficial nutrients in chocolate are magnesium and copper. A single 2-ounce bar can contribute as much as 15 percent of your daily magnesium requirement and a whopping 34 percent of your daily copper requirement. In fact, one study from the *Journal of the American Dietetic Association* estimated that as much as 9.4 percent of the U.S. required daily requirement of copper is actually supplied by chocolate!

If you're following the recommendation, and the idea of adding chocolate to your morning routine puts you in a state of shock, take a moment to assess another morning habit you may have. The average café latté is 260 calories and contains 14 grams of fat (9 grams are saturated), 21 grams of carbohydrates, and 19 grams of sugar. All things considered, dark chocolate may just have a rightful place at the breakfast table after all. You can start slowly by putting a jar of Nutella on the table, and see what happens from there (make your own Nutella-like concoction by mixing your favorite nut butter with a little melted dark chocolate and a minimal amount of natural sweetener).

Weight Gain

Recommendation

Consume high-quality dark chocolate with nuts, as needed, to curb food cravings and hunger. Eat 2–3 squares at a time, not to exceed a maximum of one 1-ounce bar per day. For extreme cases of unruly appetite, eat chocolate with ground chili peppers and drink more water. Take a 20- to 30-minute walk with friends 4 evenings per week.

Supporting Evidence

Because chocolate contains fat, it may be the most feared weapon in the diet universe. But according to an article in the *American Journal of Clinical Nutrition*, chocolate is responsible for less than 2 percent of the fat in the average diet. Most of the dietary fat actually comes from meat, dairy products, and fried foods. Recent research has uncovered a surprising collection of facts that debunk many myths about chocolate, fats, and getting fat.

As mentioned in the "Food Cravings" section, the body contains an appetite stimulant called galanin. The fat in chocolate helps curb the effects of galanin, reducing the need to eat. The cocoa powder itself is also an appetite suppressant, and, not surprisingly, numerous weight-loss products on the market actually contain cocoa powder.

Most of the fat in chocolate is considered "healthy fat," which helps raise good HDL cholesterol and lower bad LDL cholesterol. If you're counting calories, fat grams, or carbs, compare the amounts in one bar of chocolate to other snack prospects in the list below.

Chocolate also comes in very low on the glycemic index chart. Low GI foods are optimal for weight loss because they don't raise

Food	Calories	Fat Content (grams)	Carbs (grams)
1 ounce dark chocolate	143	9	17
½ cup Ben & Jerry's Chubby Hubby ice cream	350	21	33
2 Nature Valley Granola Bars	180	6	29
McDonald's Crispy Chicken Sandwich	500	26	46
Krispy Kreme glazed doughnut	210	12	22
11 Hershey's Kisses	250	4.5	9
2 dark chocolate Lindt truffles	140	12	10

blood sugar. Lower blood sugar means lower levels of insulin in the blood, and when insulin stays out of the bloodstream the fat stays off. To maintain the lowest levels of insulin, consume chocolate after meals, rather than as a snack between meals.

Nuts are included in the recommendation because the fats in nuts help satisfy the appetite. The protein and the fiber in nuts also help slow the absorption of sugar into the bloodstream, keeping blood sugar and insulin levels lower. More than one study has concluded that adding hundreds of nut calories to the diet over a six-month period does not add weight. Even when you eat enough nuts to finally induce weight gain, the actual gain is less than the expected outcome for the increased caloric intake.

If you're following the previous recommendation, you may be asking, "Why walk?" Why not hit the gym three times a week for an all-out, heavy-duty power-lifting session? Happily, research shows that light, consistent exercise is better for losing weight than is hiring a personal trainer to push you to tears every time you hit the gym. In his popular weight-loss book *Eat More, Weigh Less*, Dr. Dean Ornish recommends light exercise and confirms that strenuous workouts actually increase appetite and food intake. Less strenuous exercise works as a double positive because it allows the body to burn fat while suppressing the appetite at the same time. Walking with friends is suggested because group-supported weight-loss programs have proven to be much more successful.

If you simply can't get a raging appetite under control, consider selecting chocolates with chili peppers or spicy oils. Spicy chocolates are becoming more popular, as new companies bring original Maya and Aztec concoctions to the market, many of which include various chilies. Perhaps the svelte Maya already knew what the *British Journal of Nutrition* would report centuries later—the active compound in chilies, called capsaicin, can help reduce the appetite when consumed with meals. Subjects who consumed 10 milligrams of capsaicin before eating took in approximately 200 fewer calories per meal.

Eating chocolate will not cause excessive weight gain, but consuming too many calories and not getting enough exercise will definitely pack on the pounds. Almost anything eaten in excess will cause weight gain, whether it's fat-free ice cream, whole-grain pasta, or low-carb crackers with cheese. When you choose chocolate, the keys to weight loss are eating 70%+ dark chocolate (preferably with nuts) and keeping your consumption limited to 1 ounce per day.

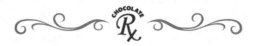

Seven

Where Do You Hide Your Chocolate?

*N*ow that you have a doctorate-level under-standing of the health benefits of chocolate, it's time to move on to some of the more entertaining aspects of the topic. Studying chocolate all day has often caused my thought processes to wander way outside the chocolate box. The results of a "Where Do You Hide Your Chocolate?" query I posted for an article were just too good not to include here. (I'd like to thank everyone who submitted responses to this survey. I couldn't use them all in this book, but I'm tempted to write another one just to share the hilarious anecdotes about hiding places that we use.)

I've edited the responses just a little, but, believe me, as you read through these you'll understand that I could not have come up with them on my own. These brilliant solutions to combat potential chocolate loss came straight from the collective creative genius of authentic chocolate hiders. I didn't even change the names to protect the innocent, and the contributors knew it. Apparently, there is no shame in hiding chocolate, and that's a good thing.

A few statistics stood out; they are summarized here for your reading pleasure:

1. We do, in fact, hide our favorite chocolates from our loved ones (or anyone else, for that matter).

2. To make up for any possible guilt over number 1, we place less-expensive "decoy" chocolate on obvious shelves to pacify others' chocolate needs and keep them from discovering the premium collection.

3. The number one hiding spot among those who responded was the freezer. If you're experiencing a chocolate emergency while at a dinner party, check here first—bottom left, under the peas and the corn. Sometimes the chocolate is in a single location; other times, you'll find it in micro-baggies spread throughout the shelves.

4. We often indulge in solitude, savoring the sweet decadence of a stolen moment with a single purpose—guiltless pleasure.

Hilarious Stories from Chocolate Hiders

Although each of us is certain that our stash is the best, a quick review of your flavor-savoring cohorts will help expand your options in the devastating event that your stockpile is ever discovered.

Joyce, sixty: A lifelong hider, Joyce began to develop her creative style in her early teens when the predicament of having to share a bedroom with her sister meant rotating the chocolate stash (tucked into a shoe box) between the center of the laundry basket and outside the bedroom window.

As Joyce matured, so did the expansion of her stash, primarily M&Ms in baggies, which extended beyond the bedroom and into every conceivable room in the house, including one pouch stapled neatly to the bottom of the couch. This spot was quite successful, in that it had never been discovered, but the installation of radiant heat some years later proved to be a carpet-destroying mishap. Not to worry—forty-four additional stashes were still intact.

Joyce maintains that over the years, the stash count has been reduced to a single baggie hanging in the pantry amid extension cords and drills. But those of us who can relate to Joyce's lifelong adventures in chocolate suspect that there's still something quite close to her pillow that she's not willing to divulge. It must be from Belgium or Switzerland.

Heidi, forty-three: Heidi, a fellow writer, uses a similar technique to mine—a bowl of chocolate chips stashed by the computer to help ease the burden of an eight-hour writing day. Come to think of it, maybe that's why we write—it's the perfect excuse to sit comfortably by a bowl of chocolate all day long.

Heidi is also one of Lindt's top customers, reportedly purchasing up to ten bags of Lindor milk chocolate truffles anytime they're on sale. Each truffle is broken into four separate bites, she insists, to make sure it constitutes the sensation of a full chocolate meal.

Her "operating" stash is kept in a small bowl in the kitchen, easily available should she be away from the computer. Obviously, ten bags of truffles would hardly fit nicely into a small mixing bowl, so the back-stock is bagged and properly disguised in the linen closet. Excellent work, Heidi.

Those wishing to discover a bit more about this chocolate-hiding cohort can check out Heidi's chocolate blog at www .heidiashworth.blogspot.com or invest in a copy of her snappy book *Miss Delacourt Speaks Her Mind*, already in the second printing since its November 2008 release. Perhaps if we all ate more chocolate, we, too, would pen brilliant stories while surrounded by our beloved chocolate chips.

Lynn, forty-four: Our hearts go out to Lynn, after she experienced the unfortunate sacrifice of several pounds of extraordinary truffles to a grazing boyfriend who mistook them for filler, as opposed to the intimate, private moments of enjoyment they're meant to be. Apparently, there are those who embrace the misguided presumption that "a truffle is a truffle is a truffle."

This is what happens when you don't hide your chocolate properly. Lynn had innocently put the truffles in the cookie jar. What kitchen-wandering man wouldn't mistake them for a low-budget cookie? This is just too obvious. I can only hope he enjoyed them with a fine-quality light lager beer.

Fortunately, Lynn assessed the folly of her ways and moved the truffles to Grandma's knitting basket before the entire lot was gone. It turned out to be an excellent alternative, given its close proximity to her reading chair, not to mention a very low possibility that the wandering grazer would stumble into Grandma's knitting. After adding a glass of red wine and a curled-up cat to the chocolate/chair combo, she quickly forgot about the missing truffles.

Michelle, thirty-nine: Michelle doesn't take chances with just one location; she goes all out with a stash in the filing cabinet at work, another in a Tupperware container at home, and chocolate mints in the freezer. To make certain the mints last as long as possible, they are individually bagged and scattered throughout the freezer. In the event of unexpected company, this strategy can help ease her stress by providing a nice chocolate surprise while she's in a frenzied search for the warehouse-size chicken potpie.

Leigh, thirty-four: Leigh wins the award for "best use of unusable glassware." Her Christmas bowls and Valentine's Day vases are not actually dusty, because they're filled with chocolate. Although it might seem simple, there's actually a bit of a balancing act involved, because the stash must be moved out of the Christmas bowls and into the Valentine's Day vase during Christmas, then back again as Valentine's Day approaches.

Yet Leigh's balancing skills are clearly intact, because she's also the mother of two small children and she owns her own business. To all of us who have walked that wire, it certainly makes sense that she needs a chocolate stash. Leigh saves her chocolate squares for her mental health time block (twenty minutes), which includes a quick peek at her favorite soap opera.

I asked myself whether a person can actually watch only twenty minutes of a soap opera. And then I realized that if you can eat only two squares of chocolate daily while raising two young children and managing your own business, you can easily tear yourself away in the midst of the average soap opera travesty.

Kathryn, age not disclosed: Kathryn represents an example of where we're all headed in this great big chocolate adventure. At the time of this writing, Katherine reported a stash of twenty-one bars in a "little" cubbyhole at her desk, although she maintains that at times there have been more. Somehow, I don't see twenty-one bars of chocolate fitting into a "little" cubbyhole, but apparently it can be done, so this is good news. I imagine one gets to a point where one learns to pack the bars perfectly to fit as many as possible into a single location.

Kathryn's response was especially close to my heart because after she listed the brands in her stash, I realized that she should probably have them in a vault, as opposed to her cubby, due to the value of her collection. And she wasn't overly snobbish about the percentage of cocoa, either. This woman just loves chocolate, from chocolate soup to chocolate-covered nuts. Her stash ranged from milk to 88% cacao, some of it pure chocolate and some infused with wasabi, chili peppers, and lemon rind.

And kudos to Kathryn, who is out there working for us. She eats half an ounce of chocolate after lunch every day and blogs about her discoveries at http://leighwantsfood.blogspot.com/search/label/chocolate. Now we don't have to work so hard to find the best!

Marlise, forty-five: Unfortunately, this woman was not able to divulge her real name for fear that her stash might be outed, leaving her chocolateless in a dire emergency. I changed both her name and her age to protect the innocent or, perhaps more appropriately, to protect her as-yet-undiscovered stash.

Before I tell you the exact location, it's important to understand that Marlise uses chocolate to manage depression and stress. She actually said that she'd have to move out if anyone discovered her hiding place, and, of course, I didn't want that to happen. (Now you begin to see why its location is level 5 security.) To make sure her chocolate doesn't suffer the same fate as that of the truffles consumed by Lynn's wandering grazer, Marlise places regular "decoy" chocolate in plain sight for her husband and son. With the naïve boys satisfied, discovery of her prized collection is far less likely.

The kicker: Although Marlise thinks this is a safe hiding place, after doing the research I can assure you that quite a large number of people hide chocolate in Tupperware under their winter sweaters. In fact, this location might come in at number two, behind "in the freezer." I'm going out on a limb here to suggest that Marlise is subconsciously worried about her stash being discovered because she actually hasn't hidden it well enough. Perhaps she'll be prepared to use her real name without fear of discovery after reading this section.

Stacie, age not disclosed: Stacie uses the strategy "when the going gets tough, the tough eat their chocolate stash." She is the mother of three small children and has a chocolate-obsessed husband, so you can only imagine the wall of potential conspiracy she is up against to locate a safe place for her chocolate. But Stacie's creativity runs deep, ensuring that her chocolate will be safe for decades. In fact, she may single-handedly own the top three spots in the world.

1. In the sanitary napkin box in the bathroom closet. True brilliance, not to mention perfectly appropriate for the occasion.

2. In the box that contains her wedding album. Where else could you possibly hide chocolate from a chocolate-obsessed husband? I've personally never seen a man reminisce through a wedding album, and I'd be willing to bet money that it's happened less than ten times throughout history. Very clever.

3. In a shoe box at the top of her closet. After all, one can truly only expect to find an old pair of ladies' shoes there, right?

Diana, forty-five: Diana didn't actually disclose the exact location of her stash, although she did tell a very sweet story about how she and her six-year-old daughter fight over the stash (okay, "fight" might be a bit dramatic). She mentioned that she keeps a large bag of chocolate chips in the pantry with the baking goods—"decoy" chocolate, I presume.

I had to include this story because it reminds me of what happens when you ask your kids what they've been doing, and instead of answering, they ask you how your day was. It's not that they really care how it was—it's simply that they don't want to tell you what they've been doing. Likewise, when a hider won't anonymously divulge where she is hiding something, it's safe to say we have a true hider.

Tracy, forty-three: Tracy is a freezer hider, but considering that she's the mom of two teenage sons, she definitely doesn't have to worry that they'll be looking in there anytime soon. In fact, they may not open the freezer until their midthirties, when their wives leave home for the first time on a business trip. Simplicity can be a beautiful thing, and Tracy has capitalized on it nicely.

Actually, there's a little more to her story that's worth pointing out. Tracy discovered that although her sons inherited her brown hair and brown eyes (she suspects this is where their love of chocolate stems from), they did not inherit her love of vegetables. It's highly unlikely that her sons would ever think to even touch a bag of peas or corn, much less move them, unless, of course, they were sitting on top of half a gallon of chocolate ice cream.

Tracy is optimizing a technique I call "using idiosyncrasy to your favor." If you know your potential targets would never cook anything, a kitchen-focused location is destined for success. Your kids or husband won't wash clothes? The laundry room. Not a tea drinker? The tea canister. Not a knitter? The knitting basket. Well, you get the point.

Christy, twenty-eight: "Guilty pleasure" is a term often associated with chocolate indulgence (although, hopefully, not after people read this book), and Christy is the quintessential example of this. She hides her chocolate in her workout drawer, right next to her gym clothes, requiring her to carefully assess just exactly how badly she wants her chocolate. In case the answer is very badly, she keeps two different bags flattened neatly under the shorts and the T-shirts. This keeps her options open, while giving her enough room to stow both the chocolate and the clothes and still close the drawer easily.

Krista, forty-five: Discipline is the order of the day when you keep chocolate in the vicinity, and Krista has plenty of it. She keeps the good stuff (imported) on the bottom shelf of her pantry, under the elegant table linens, demonstrating excellent use of little-used household items. She claims to venture there several times a week, where she rotates between a collection of Valrhona, Côte d'Or, and Toblerone. She claims that she eats only small amounts of the best chocolate—an excellent strategy for anyone considering a chocolate-hiding program.

Krista also uses "decoy" chocolate to keep the hounds at bay, although she calls it "strawman" chocolate. Whichever term you decide to use, it's an excellent idea and should be employed by every genuine chocolate hider.

Ruth, fifty-five: Ruth is a self-proclaimed novice chocolate hider, and it appears that she hides it from herself. As a novice, she's not had the opportunity to experience having her favorite chocolate around the house on a regular basis, so she puts it in unusual places that she's not likely to see, hoping she'll actually skip a day or two between indulgences.

Fortunately, she eats dark chocolate with nuts, one of the healthiest options. So, even if she goes overboard and eats more than one piece per day, she's still in good hands with her chocolate choice. She spreads the chocolates out among file drawers around the house, in her attempt to restrict herself to one piece per day.

To the lifelong hider, this concept may seem simply incomprehensible. Hide chocolate from ourselves? Are you kidding? But let's be gentle with the newbies, because there are bound to be more of them as time progresses. We must band together and help them bridge the gap between the love of chocolate and self-discipline.

Lucy, age not disclosed: Like Heidi, Lucy is another fellow writer tucked away behind the computer with a lifesaving chocolate stash. The title of her book *If Mama Don't Laugh, It Ain't Funny* is a perfect explanation of her humorous response to my query. Hiding place number one is the pantry, but, as the mother of four kids, she found that she herself has to hide in the pantry to eat it. So her hiding spot is all accommodating—large enough for both her and the chocolate at the same time.

The pantry seems like an obvious place, of course. Who wouldn't look there for chocolate? But a simple sticky note has solved the problem of discovery: "Saved for recipe." Amazingly, no one has caught on yet, so you may want to try this at your house.

At the office, her chocolate is carefully nestled between a few rustled papers in a lower desk drawer. Apparently, she works in an office of chocolate-loving women. Should she miss a day due to illness, her entire stash could be wiped out. The lower-drawer option works perfectly because she can easily bend down to attend to papers while indulging in the necessary bite, completely unnoticed.

One final place—her roadside emergency stash in the car. Obviously, this is a questionable location due to the probability of a sunny day, and Lucy admitted that there have been some episodes of melting. If you've just been pulled over for speeding, however, and your kids are late for soccer, the baby is crying, and your hair is in rollers, the fact that your car–chocolate stash might have melted hardly seems worth considering. Just have a napkin and a mirror handy.

Heather, thirty-eight: Heather has the unique requirement of preferring to eat her chocolate at room temperature. To keep her chocolate consumption in check, she stashes her collection in the freezer. When she wants a little chocolate, it's not a snap decision for her, because she must wait until it thaws out.

I've never actually waited until chocolate thaws before eating it, so I'm not exactly sure how long it takes to go from a solid freeze to room temperature. Yet it appears to work for Heather, who maintains that she is a successful recovering chocoholic, and this technique suits her perfectly. I may try it someday just to see how long it takes, but I'd have to eat a different piece of chocolate while I waited.

Gerette, thirty-nine: Another queen of discipline, Gerette is actually able to limit herself to one piece of Godiva per day. She keeps it stashed in one of the drawers in the kitchen island. As such, we must presume that Gerette does most of the cooking in her house, because this seems like a readily available location. But read on, because this is only part of her clever program.

Gerette also shared her purchasing technique, which involves buying on-sale Godiva only with cash to avoid a paper trail. It's quite good planning, because if her husband saw Godiva on the credit card bill, it wouldn't take him long to discover her stash. As it is now, he never thinks to look for it. She also decided that the $150 box should not be purchased, even at half off, because it couldn't be hidden adequately in the drawer. This woman has clearly come to know her chocolate.

Paula, forty-four: Scrapbooking has been all the rage for quite some time, yet there are people who have no idea why. Paula is not one of them. Not only is an entire room in her house dedicated to scrapbooking, but her scrapbook-questioning family dare not enter the room.

Scrapbookers know exactly what I'm talking about, and you're probably laughing now. I can't speak from personal experience, but my sister is part of the clan, so I faithfully stand by the words. Of course, it makes sense that an ardent scrapbooker would hide her chocolate in the off-limits room as well. Paula says she waits until everyone is gone for the day, then steals away into the room for her savored indulgence. If they only knew what else was in there!

Her backup stash is equally well-concealed: in her underwear drawer. Admittedly, not too many people are going to rummage around in there, either. Between the scrapbook room and the underwear drawer, Paula's chocolate will most likely remain available to her for decades, possibly even a century.

Teresa, forty-eight: This was one of the most unique hiding places of all of those divulged, though apparently not as well thought out as Teresa might have originally intended.

An unexpectedly helpful husband stumbled on the laundry-room stash after inadvertently tossing a load of freshly washed clothes into the dryer. Teresa, who had stashed an extra piece of chocolate cake in the dryer earlier, knew she was busted when he wandered out of the laundry room and posed the question, "Do we have a problem?" She didn't mention exactly how she answered, but I imagine that a fairly spirited discussion ensued, especially considering that he had run the dryer before discovering her covert operation.

I've never actually run a piece of chocolate cake through the dryer—or even a simple chocolate bar, for that matter. After thinking it through, it occurred to me that the dryer might not fare that well under those circumstances, much less the clothes. Normally, I wouldn't intervene in this type of personal issue, but unless you're single and not prone to absentmindedness, this is probably not an ideal strategy.

Karen, forty-three: This could be the most feared event in a hider's life: a stash is discovered. The hider is outed. Devastation sets in. She asks herself the heart-pounding question—What do I do now?

Fellow hider Karen took the discovery in stride. After realizing that her husband was tapping into her stash, she emptied the contents and filled the former location with kitty kibble. A thoughtful note was placed on top, with a simple message: "Ha! Caught you!"

Given this lighthearted and humorous response, it's safe to presume that the couple is still married and that Karen's new hiding place will never, ever be discovered. Other hiders might not have taken to the discovery with such mild amusement, but perhaps we could all learn from this strategy.

Valerie, age not disclosed: Valerie owns Chicago Chocolate Tours (www.ChicagoChocolateTours.com), so by extreme necessity she must have an extraordinary place for her premium reserve or it's bound to be discovered by her staff, if not her customers. Valerie had really thought through the details, defining exactly what qualities an ideal hiding place should have. In her own words: "One that is memorable to you, so that you don't forget where you put the magic stuff, yet counterintuitive so that anybody snooping around won't stumble onto your stash, and also safe for the chocolate, so that it won't pick up smells from other foods or materials, and not too hot or too cold."

Her special place? Amid the pile of bills. Not only will no one be rummaging through your bills, but when *you're* rummaging through them, you'll actually find something enjoyable. The only downside I could see to this strategy is that if you pay all of your bills right when they come in, your stack won't be big enough to cover your stash. So, if you're one of these prompt people (there may be only a handful of them in the world), I guess this option won't work for you.

Virginia, age not disclosed: A second-generation hider, Virginia learned her doctorate-level hiding skills from her mother, whom she claims was a highly skilled hider. Virginia also honed her hiding talent out of necessity, because she's the mother of three die-hard candy-snooping kids. Like Michelle, Virginia doesn't take chances with a single-stash location. She hides in her clean socks, behind the books, at the bottom of the tampon box, in the sewing basket, in the files of the filing cabinet, under the mattress, in her bathrobe pocket, and in the travel mugs in the kitchen.

You might think this would be enough, but not so. Virginia has taken her hiding to extremes by keeping her larger and more expensive brands in a lockbox that isn't only locked—it's also hidden under the bed. She didn't mention where she'd hidden the key, but it's safe to assume that it's locked up as well. If chocolate hiding is ever added as an Olympic sport, I suspect we'll see Virginia giving a strong run for the gold.

Caroline, thirty-one: Caroline's unique hiding twist is akin to teaching an old dog new tricks. The necessity for Caroline's stash stems from her having a job in the food industry at Behind the Burner (www.BehindtheBurner.com). She's constantly surrounded not only by food samples of all kinds but also by foodies of every type, so, of course, any self-respecting chocolate stash is in serious jeopardy of quickly disappearing.

I was surprised that Caroline decided to divulge the location of her stash because in the event that her cohorts read this book, she'll have to come up with another brilliant place. Yet her idea is so good, it would almost be a crime not to share it, so she must have another spot in mind already.

Caroline hides chocolate in the office fridge, but her strategy is unique because she knows it will be viewed by many eyes. She places her stash in an unattractive bag from an inconspicuous café, crumpling it in the proper manner to ensure its resemblance to three-week-old leftovers. Of course, a gorgeous bag from the local chocolate shop would garner far too much attention, but her simple almost-trash plan works perfectly. Most people would never dream of looking in a beat-to-shreds old bag for a stash of exquisite chocolate. As such, her stash is safe.

Kat, age not disclosed: Kat has a reverse-hiding situation at her house. Her kids have to hide their chocolate from her. She has four boys (now we understand why Kat likes chocolate so much), and they discovered the hard way that no chocolate left out in the open is safe. After a birthday party, one of the younger tots errantly left his chocolate-laden goody bag on the table. Chores are so much easier to do when you're eating chocolate, and, of course, Kat had plenty of work to do with four boys running amok.

When her son came home later to retrieve the newly emptied bag, he ran to his mother and demanded to know whether she'd eaten the goods. After her sheepish admittance, he burst into tears. Kat had to stifle a laugh when she heard her older boy reprimand his younger brother by saying, "Luke, you *know* you can't leave chocolate lying around in this house! If she sees it, she's gonna eat it!" So you see, it wasn't her fault after all.

Cynthia, age not disclosed: Cynthia contributed on behalf of her father, whom she calls a lifelong chocoholic. Because he suffered from diabetes and was heavier than would be considered healthy, Cynthia attempted to get him on track with a month-long program at a live-in health facility. She took her children for a visit, noting with interest that her father had brought his piggy bank. But because men often do strange things, she put it out of her mind.

Sometime after they'd left, she learned from her daughter (who had been sworn to secrecy by her grandfather) that the piggy bank was filled with chocolate coins, rather than real money. Apparently, despite the fact that her father was exercising and eating perfectly all day, he was deep into the piggy bank in the evening.

Clearly touched by her grandfather's passion for chocolate, Cynthia's daughter is now (years later) studying to be a chocolatier. I've always suspected that there's something in the gene pool, and research seems to conclude that this very well could be the case.

Rebecca, thirty: Rebecca uses a technique I call "referred chocolate hiding," because she doesn't directly hide it herself. She requires an associate-in-hiding, and in this case, it's her beloved husband. Bless him for keeping her from the chocolate "demons," as she calls them, which makes me suspect that she may be a novice hider who hasn't fully developed her self-discipline (in time, though, she will).

In this case, Rebecca actually knows where the stash is, but she has no idea how to gain access because it's locked in the gun safe, and only her husband knows the combination. I tried to imagine what it would be like to see a gun every time I visited my chocolate stash and decided that it might not be an ideal situation, at least for me, because occasionally I'm in pursuit of the stash while in a highly questionable mood. Yet because Rebecca does not know the combination, this probably isn't an issue for her.

Sheila, age not disclosed: Not only are you going to love Sheila, but you'll want to know the name of her doctor, too. I'm dubbing her the "chocolate angel" because she sent me the most selfless response I've received. She has three caches (as she calls them), one of which is in the bottom drawer of her desk at work. An obvious place, but it doesn't matter to her because she shares her chocolate with everyone in the office (sorry, workplace not revealed). Her officemates renamed her collection "Emergency Truffles."

Her second stash is in a chest of living-room drawers. After a personal tragedy struck, her doctor recommended that she have a piece of good-quality dark chocolate and a shot of tequila each evening to help her combat depression. She followed the prescription for eighteen months, after which she dropped the tequila (fortunately) and continued with the chocolate (fortunately again).

Cache number three is the roadside emergency box. This brings to mind the previous car–chocolate stasher and the possibility of finding yourself with a flat on a warm day. As previously noted, include a napkin and a mirror with the car stash, and all is well.

I'm starting a movement for all chocolate hiders to embrace Sheila's pay-it-forward plan. Give it away, and it will come back to you, probably when you need it most. You'll be sitting at your desk, having lost a big client or pouting about a relationship gone awry, or maybe you simply broke a nail on a new manicure.

Someone will walk up to you with a bar of organic dark chocolate with tart dried cherries and Vietnamese cinnamon, and suddenly the world will look different.

Like me, you may have realized that with the exception of undisclosed ages, most of the respondents are women in their thirties and forties. Although this is only a small sample of the responses I pored through, this statistic held true for all of them. The researcher in me was piqued, so I developed a few theories about this potential anomaly for consideration:

- We've hit the age of "I don't care. I'm going to do what I want." Guilt-free chocolate enjoyment is now the norm, not the exception.

- Women are the only people who are actually doing any reading and query answering on the Internet. Kids are watching YouTube and downloading songs onto their iTouch, and men are vacillating among gambling, sports, and questionable Web sites.

- We want to see our stashes in writing somewhere, thereby validating their existence while keeping the true location a secret.

- And finally, we've formed a Worldwide Hiders Alliance, and we're attempting to connect with our herd.

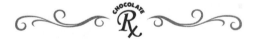

Eight

Chocolate and Wine Pairing

P UNTIL A COUPLE of years ago, no one ever really thought about enjoying chocolate and wine together. Fortunately, it makes complete sense to people who have a passion for both. So when the first version of *The Chocolate Therapist* led to my teaching classes about chocolate and wine, the next step—creating a written guide—was a natural.

I've done hundreds of pairings of wines and chocolates from all over the world. I've matched them by country, flavor, bean, region, contrast, infusion, nuance, body, chocolate percentage, custom creation—every category you can possibly imagine. I've paired them in classes, on cruises, at social gatherings, in a bar, with friends, with strangers, or just because. The research was often painstaking—so many wines and chocolates, day after day. It took a modicum of self-discipline to keep to the recommended maximum, yet somehow I didn't find it too taxing. Occasionally, I forced my students to step up as guinea pigs, but no one complained much.

Because *The Chocolate Therapist* is about healthy chocolate, the pairings are not a carte-blanche selection of unhealthy decadent desserts. Most are unique and eclectic recipes that are designed to promote health, as well as intrigue the palate. This section is not only about how to pair chocolate and wine but also about how to enjoy chocolate with infusions that pair wonderfully with wine while promoting optimal health as well. Not every pairing epitomizes a perfectly healthy option, but at least one of the chocolate pairings with every wine can be enjoyed for health, as well as for flavor.

Wine and Health News Breaks

The news about red wine and heart health first came out in 1991 on *60 Minutes*. The phenomenon was called the "French Paradox," and the show focused on the fact that the French, who drink considerably more wine than Americans do, have much lower levels of heart disease. The story ran twice that year, and Americans responded by increasing their purchases of red wine the following year by 39 percent. *This* is how we embrace a health trend.

Similar information is now being released about chocolate. Although we don't yet see medical professionals encouraging us to eat chocolate every day, some doctors and dieticians are suggesting an ounce per day for health. As more research unveils the health benefits of dark chocolate, we're likely to see more recommendations to eat specifically dark chocolate as well.

Similarities between Chocolate and Wine

Chocolate and wine share many of the same qualities when it comes to pairing and tasting, the first of which is that both are fruits. We've known this about wine for centuries, but many people don't realize that chocolate is also made from a fruit.

The processing of chocolate and wine is also very similar. Cocoa processing involves the harvest, splitting the pods, scooping the beans from the pods, fermenting, roasting, winnowing the shells, and finally grinding the beans into a thick chocolate soup called chocolate liquor—the basis of all things chocolate.

Wine starts with the harvest, the crushing of the grapes, fermentation, blending (depending on the wine being produced), aging, and bottling into the finished product. The reason wine and chocolate are so rich in antioxidants is that both are made from the ground seeds of a fruit tree. One could argue that producing chocolate is a bit more labor-intensive than making wine, but many elements are the same.

More similarities between the two are found in their growing regions. Like wine, chocolate (called cacao before processing) also comes from regions all over the world. Cacao requires a hot, humid environment and grows in a band approximately 20 degrees north and south of the equator. Wine grows from about 20 to 60 degrees north and south of the equator, just outside the band of cacao growing. Because of this, wine grows in an estimated sixty countries, whereas only thirty-three countries currently grow cacao.

Within countries, cacao tree types change from region to region, and the taste of the beans also changes, just as grapes do. The trees pick up the nuances of the land and pass their flavors into the cacao beans. Similar characteristics are found in grape vines as well. There are more than two hundred flavor compounds in wine and more than four hundred in chocolate, making the possible combinations virtually unlimited.

How to Eat Chocolate Properly

Eating chocolate "properly" is an important step in appreciating a good pairing. Most people eat far too fast, so the intent of this section is to get you to slow down. There's simply no way to discover more than four hundred flavor compounds if the chocolate is in and out of your mouth in less than ten seconds. Food should arrive in your stomach in liquid form—how often does that actually happen?

You can review chapter 5 for the intricate details on proper chocolate tasting. Once you slow down and truly enjoy the chocolate, you'll be able to investigate brands you've been eating from an entirely new perspective (even the off-the-shelf bars you grab as you fly through the grocery store).

It's easier to identify flavors when they're listed in front of you. To help train your palate, the Chocolate Wheel of Flavor, developed by Rose Potts of Blommer Chocolate Company, is included on the next page. Once you have a piece of chocolate melted in your mouth thoroughly, check the wheel to help you uncover the mysteries. It seems obvious that you would know what you're tasting, but sometimes you won't remember a flavor until you see its name. With the wheel, you'll have dozens of choices in front of you.

Blommer Chocolate was founded in 1939 and is still family owned and operated. It's North America's largest cocoa-bean processor and chocolate manufacturer and serves customers around the world.

Blommer Chocolate Wheel of Flavor

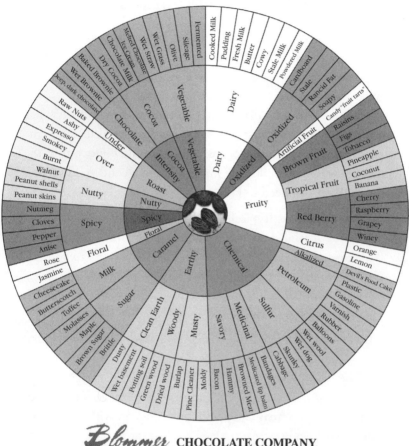

Blommer CHOCOLATE COMPANY

East Greenville, PA • Chicago, IL • Union City, CA • Campbellford, Ontario

This chart will help train your palate until you become
a discerning connoisseur of chocolate.

The company manufactures a broad array of chocolate, cocoa powder, and specialty coatings, including a signature organic line of chocolates. Blommer Chocolate also makes high-end cocoas formulated for the confectionary, baking, and dairy industries. For your own copy of the copyrighted flavor wheel, contact Blommer through its Web site, www.blommer.com.

Selecting the Proper Wineglass

The next step is a brief education on how to enjoy wine from the correct glass. It's not imperative to have the precise glass described here, of course, but having the knowledge of the best choice gives you an option if you want to use it.

Anyone who has dined in the twenty-first century has undoubtedly noticed that various wines are served in different-shaped glasses. Entire classes are devoted to the topic, but in the interest of time, the following information is a condensed version of everything you need to know.

White wine glass: Typically smaller than a red wine glass for the purpose of concentrating the bouquet (or smell) in the glass. Make sure to breathe in the aromas before you sip, to appreciate the wine from this glass. The wineglass is also slightly closed at the top to help maintain the temperature of the wine, which is primarily served chilled.

Red wine glass: The larger, balloon-shaped glass helps oxidize the wine once it's out of the bottle, adding flavor and bouquet to the overall experience. Swirling the wine in the glass helps release the aromas. Take care not to get too overzealous in your churning or you may end up dousing your date with wine (however, this is an excellent strategy if you want to leave early).

Champagne glass: The long fluted shape serves two purposes—it helps keep the Champagne cool and also releases the bubbles from a single point. Although bubble-watching can offer stimulating entertainment at a boring dinner party, its real purpose is to preserve the Champagne just a bit longer, if you haven't already chugged it.

Port glass: The primary reason for the smaller size of this glass is to allow you to enjoy a full glass while drinking a smaller amount of port. Due to the unusual expense of port, the smaller glass is a good concept for dining establishments but not such a good value for the consumer. On a positive note, considering the higher alcohol content of port, along with the likelihood that you'll be drinking it toward the end of the evening, the smaller glass also serves as protection against the possibility of overindulging.

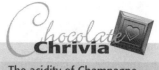

Chocolate Chrivia

The acidity of Champagne and sparkling wines can give chocolate a tart taste. For best results, pair your dark chocolate with red wine.

How to Taste Wine

Just as with chocolate, there are published guidelines on how to taste wine properly. If you're like most people, you've been drinking wine without much consideration for years, but change is good and the time is now.

Ideally, your wine should be poured into the proper glass for maximum flavor and aroma. In case you skipped that section, it's right before this one and takes less than two minutes to read.

Red wine should be opened before you serve it to help aerate the wine, although not much happens in that regard unless it's poured into a decanter. To really release the aromas and aerate the wine, pour it into a larger container. White wine is normally served chilled and occasionally served at room temperature.

Next, pour the wine into the glass and observe the color. Some people prefer to hold a white cloth or napkin to the back of the glass to get a true assessment of color. The depth of the color can indicate the intensity of the flavor.

Swirl the wine in the glass to help release its aroma and nuances. While it runs back down the side of the glass, note the viscosity. If you see thin streams of wine running down the glass, it's said to have "legs." Take a long sniff or two to excite your olfactory glands and help wake up your taste buds. Smell is accountable for as much as 90 percent of everything you taste, so it's in your best interest to take time for this step.

Next, take a small sip of the wine, but don't swallow immediately. Keep it in your mouth and swirl it around your tongue, looking for flavor notes such as fruit, oak, earth, mineral, sweet, sour, bitter, and salty. Observe the texture—is it smooth, light, full, or delicate?

Try taking a breath though your nose with the wine still in your mouth. Think carefully about this procedure because taking a breath while swallowing could cause some problems. The key, of course, is not to swallow exactly at the same time that you're breathing.

The last step, finally, is to swallow. But your job isn't finished! How long does the flavor last? What are the lingering nuances? Is it sweet, acidic, robust, tannic, or strong in alcohol? There are so many things to consider. You may have to take another sip to get it right.

To help with flavor identification, see the Wine Aroma Wheel by Ann Noble on the next page. Having the flavors at your fingertips can help you determine the wine's exact essences and aromas. The strategy here is the same as the Chocolate Flavor Wheel: once you have the wine in your mouth, look at the different flavors on the wheel to help discern what you taste.

Putting It All Together

People always ask me which comes first when pairing—the wine or the chocolate? Personally, I prefer to put the chocolate in my mouth first, taking special care to follow the "Proper Chocolate

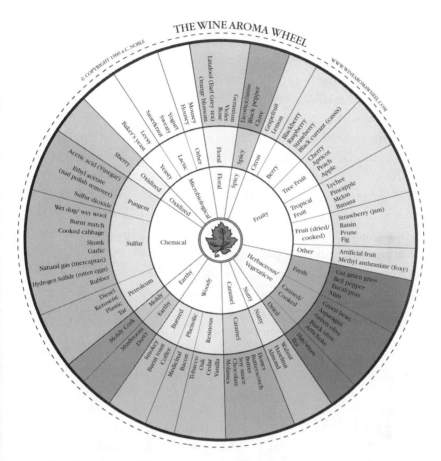

The Wine Aroma Wheel is the ultimate reference when discovering the flavors in wine.* Copyright © A. C. Noble, 1990, 2002.

Consumption" instructions in chapter 5. This gives the chocolate a chance to melt before you add the wine. If the wine is cool, it can lower the temperature of your mouth and make melting more challenging.

---

* Laminated wheels can be purchased at retail and wholesale prices on Ann Noble's Web site at www.WineAromaWheel.com. The wheel is also available in French, Italian, Spanish, Norwegian, Danish, and Swedish.

As you're assessing the chocolate, pour about a third of a glass of wine. Swirl the wine in the glass and take short sniffs, as reviewed in "How to Taste Wine." Take a small sip and swish the wine around with the chocolate so that the two mingle together. Note how the flavors of the chocolate have changed. Some of the flavors will be accentuated by the wine; others will be covered up. Sometimes the wine is too strong for the chocolate, or the chocolate may be too strong for the wine. You're looking for balance. The perfect pairing accentuates both the wine and the chocolate.

After you've paired the wine and the chocolate in this order, reverse the process and drink the wine first, followed by eating the chocolate. Remember to go slowly—smell the wine . . . take a small sip and note the flavors . . . add the chocolate . . . note how the flavors of both the chocolate and the wine change. If you rush, this takes away from the process, and you'll miss quite a few of the flavors. Remember, there are more than six hundred flavors between the chocolate and the wine!

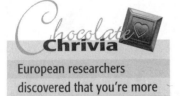

Chrivia

European researchers discovered that you're more likely to catch a mouse with chocolate than with cheese.

Before you switch to the next pairing, cleanse your palate with bland crackers or water. A salt-free table cracker works well because salt changes the palate considerably. It's also best to drink room-temperature water to keep your mouth warm.

Red Wine and Chocolate Pairings

For pairing purposes, it's important to note that wines are generally classified into three different body types—light, medium, and full. A light-bodied wine is in and out of your mouth quickly, and you taste it only while it's in your mouth. It's also typically lighter in color, and you can see through it. Lighter reds generally have higher acidity levels and are best drunk when relatively young. Open a bottle of light-bodied red, and you'll want to finish the bottle immediately. Examples of lighter reds include pinot noir, gamay, Beaujolais, and an occasional merlot.

A medium-bodied wine lingers a while after you've swallowed it, allowing you to assess the taste and the aftertaste longer than the lighter wines. It's generally a moderate shade of red or burgundy. It contains more tannins than the lighter reds, although you'll still want to enjoy this wine right after opening the bottle. Leave it around longer than four days, and most of the flavor will be gone. To stretch out its life, put it in the refrigerator to help stop oxidation, as well as the buildup of mold. Examples of medium-bodied wines include merlot, Sangiovese, and occasionally zinfandel, although each of these wines can be full-bodied as well.

Full-bodied wine flavors last long after the wine has been swallowed and offer changing taste sensations on the finish. The color is deep and rich—not something that can easily be gazed through. The fullest wines have the greatest level of tannins. Full-bodied wines also last a little longer—after two days, you may discover flavors you didn't notice on opening. Examples of full-bodied wines include cabernet sauvignon, cabernet franc, and Shiraz.

The details provided for each wine in the pairing section that follows are general, and you won't taste every flavor listed for each wine. Flavors depend on many elements, such as growing regions, production techniques, and the average temperature during the growing season. The following are flavors you "may" find in each wine. They're included here because having a list of flavors will help you discern nuances you might not otherwise be able to identify. It will also help you pair the chocolates more appropriately.

All recipes identified by an asterisk can be found in chapter 9, in this book.

To create your own versions of many of the concoctions in this section, see the first section of chapter 9 and learn how to microwave your own chocolate. And there's no need to limit your pairings to those provided here—go wild with your own, too!

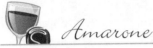

Amarone

Grapes used to make: Corvina, Rondinella, Sangiovese, Molinara

Regions grown in: Italy/Veneto

Body: Full-bodied, soft tannins, higher alcohol, often dry, long flavor

Flavors: Dried fruit, ripe wild berries, candied fruit, chocolate, charcoal, cinnamon, baked cherries, smoke, truffle, sweet, port, earth

Notes: Whatever you're serving, make sure it's powerful enough to withstand the strength of this popular Italian wine. It's a great wine for foods with bold tastes; try a dark chocolate mole sauce with raspberries over chicken.

Adventurous Chocolate Pairings

Conservative: Dark chocolate cherry truffle

Edgy: 70% melted dark chocolate, dried blueberries, and two drops of vanilla

Gone wild: Dark chocolate–covered pecans dipped in Raspberry/Pomegranate Puree*

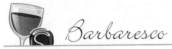

Barbaresco

Grapes used to make: Nebbiolo

Regions grown in: Italy/Piedmont

Body: Medium- to full-bodied, bold, spicy, tannic, elegant, good balance, long on palate; a powerful wine that holds up well with bold flavors

Flavors: Earthy, fig, nut, leather, tar, mushroom, vanilla, cinnamon, plum, raspberry, black cherry, violet, truffle, sweet red fruit, licorice, menthol, mineral, tar, spice

Notes: The hallmark flavors of Barbaresco are violet and truffles, so a violet truffle becomes the obvious choice when pairing with chocolate. If you don't know where to buy a violet truffle, try Wild Women Truffles (www.WildWomenTruffles .com). Prepare for the taste-tantalizing brilliance of Kathy and Debbie's world-renowned truffles.

Adventurous Chocolate Pairings

Conservative: Single-origin Ecuadorian chocolate, known for its heavy anise flavor

Edgy: Violet truffles, as mentioned above

Gone wild: Dark chocolate–covered figs sprinkled with sesame seeds

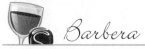

Barbera

Grapes used to make: Nebbiolo

Regions grown in: Italy/Piedmont, California

Body: Medium-bodied, smooth, low tannins with high acidity

Flavors: Blackberries, plums, black pepper, cinnamon, vanilla, smoke, milk chocolate, cedar, toasted oak, mineral, spice, cherry, raspberry, earth

Notes: This wine is particularly suited to Mediterranean foods, making it ideal for pairing with fruits from the same region, such as red currants, cranberries, and gooseberries.

Adventurous Chocolate Pairings

> **Conservative**: Milk and dark chocolate together, either melted and lightly swirled or a bite of each together
>
> **Edgy**: 70% dark chocolate with chili peppers
>
> **Gone wild**: Double Dark Chocolate Brownies* topped with fresh blackberries, raspberries, and melted dark mint chocolate

 Barolo

Grapes used to make: Nebbiolo

Grown in: Italy/Piedmont, California

Body: Rich, medium- to full-bodied, heavy, high alcohol content, higher tannins when young

Flavors: Black cherry, leather, tar, earthy, mushroom, chocolate, floral, roses, herbs, wood, hazelnut, berries, coconut, vanilla, raspberry, spicy, oregano, tobacco, anise, smoke, violet, rose

Notes: Salt has a tendency to make tannic wines slightly sweeter, hence the "Edgy" recommendation for a bit of sea salt with the pairing. Who better than you to determine whether this adventure is one worth repeating?

Adventurous Chocolate Pairings

> **Conservative**: Dark chocolate infused with rose (try Chocopologie at www.knipschildt.net/chba.html)
>
> **Edgy**: Dark chocolate coconut haystack dusted with sea salt
>
> **Gone wild**: Dried mangos dipped in melted 75% dark single-origin Ivory Coast chocolate with a drop of clove oil

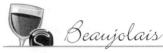

Beaujolais

Grapes used to make: Gamay

Regions grown in: France/Burgundy region of Beaujolais, Switzerland

Body: Light body, low tannins, refreshing

Flavors: Berries, cherries, blackberries, strawberries, black currants, cedar, earth, leather, floral

Beaujolais: Made from 100% gamay grapes, generally light and fruity

Beaujolais Nouveau: The lightest, fruitiest, and youngest of the Beaujolais family. The time from harvest to retail is often less than two months. Once you open the bottle, consume it within hours, or there will hardly be anything left to taste.

Beaujolais Villages: A step up from Nouveau, Beaujolais Villages wines are produced in regions known to grow higher-quality grapes.

Beaujolais Cru: The best Beaujolais money can buy. Look for the word *Cru* on the label.

Notes: When considering chocolate, go for the lighter dark chocolate, such as 45 to 55% dark with fruity and/or nutty nuances. Very dark chocolate will bury the wine, and you'll end up with bitterness. Also note that citrus and cream flavors can clash with Beaujolais.

Adventurous Chocolate Pairings

Conservative: 55% dark chocolate with raspberries

Edgy: Melted 45% dark chocolate with dried cherries and two drops of vanilla

Gone wild: Sliced tart green apples dipped in a blend of melted cheddar cheese and 55% dark Ecuadorian chocolate

 Bordeaux

Grapes used to make: Generally a combination of many different grapes, including cabernet sauvignon, merlot, cabernet franc, Malbec, and Petit Verdot

Regions grown: France/Bordeaux, Italy

Body: Medium- to full-bodied, soft to moderate tannins, smooth

Flavors: Oak, blackberry, Indian spices, licorice, green olive, dark olive, plum, mineral, floral, jammy, cherry, strawberry, smoke, earth, cassis, black currant, dried herbs, toast, vanilla, cedar, roasted coffee, mocha, cola

Notes: Bordeaux is any wine produced in the Bordeaux region of France, so narrowing the field of flavors and grapes is almost impossible. Read the labels to determine the flavors of your Bordeaux, then select the chocolate accordingly.

Adventurous Chocolate Pairings

Conservative: Dark chocolate with black currants

Edgy: Chocolate-covered espresso beans

Gone wild: Chocolate-covered black licorice sprinkled with cinnamon

 Brunello

Grapes used to make: Brunello, Sangiovese

Regions grown: Italy/Tuscany

Body: Full-bodied, generally longer on finish, strength in tannins

Flavors: Blackberry, vanilla, Indian spices, currant, toasted oak, cherry, berry, anise, menthol, cedar, earth, tea, raspberry, smoke, chocolate truffles, black mushrooms, spicy, blueberry, plums, prunes, tar, chestnuts

Notes: Brunello is the signature wine of Italy's Montalcino region, considered by some to be one of Italy's best wines. Unexpected bold flavors and aromas keep the chocolate pairing options wide open for negotiation, so if you don't see something that piques your palate here, investigate a collection of your own concoctions.

Adventurous Chocolate Pairings

Conservative: Raspberry Dark Chocolate Truffles*

Edgy: Fresh blueberries dipped in melted dark chocolate with a pinch of chili pepper

Gone wild: Dark chocolate with chopped hazelnuts and pumpkin seeds; sprinkling of curry optional

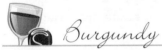 *Burgundy*

Grapes used to make: Pinot noir; less expensive wines may also include gamay

Region grown in: France/Burgundy

Body: Medium to full-bodied, full ripe tannins, long finish

Flavors: Raspberries, plums, spice, floral, blackberry, cherry, leather, earthiness, pomegranate, flowers, vanilla, chocolate, apple, pineapple, banana, mayflower, hazelnut

Notes: The Burgundy region in France produces both red and white wines. A true red Burgundy is made only from the pinot noir grape, although less expensive versions may include gamay grapes as well. Blends are considered second-class to the great Burgundies of the region.

Adventurous Chocolate Pairings

Conservative: Sea salt pretzels dipped in dark chocolate

Edgy: Pomegranate and Cinnamon Double Dark Chocolate Brownies*

Gone wild: Tart Apple/Blackberry Pie* with Dark Vanilla Chocolate Drizzle* and chopped hazelnuts

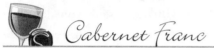 *Cabernet Franc*

Grapes used to make: Cabernet franc, cabernet sauvignon, merlot

Regions grown in: France/Bordeaux and the Loire Valley, California/Napa Valley, Washington

Body: Medium- to full-bodied, gentle tannins, high acidity

Flavors: Raspberries, cherries, cinnamon, plum, tea, cedar, spicy, green peppers, cocoa powder, savory, flowers, earthy, tarragon, dried cherry, coffee, anise, bay, herbs, white pepper, vanilla, tobacco leaf, allspice, clove, Heath bar, cream, raspberry, currant, blackberry, mineral

Notes: Cabernet franc is generally blended with the two grapes mentioned above, although it's possible to find wine made from cabernet franc grapes alone. This versatile wine often contains chocolate notes on the finish, making it a natural for pairing.

Adventurous Chocolate Pairings

Conservative: Berried in Chocolate—cherries, raspberries, and cranberries in dark chocolate (available at www .TheChocolateTherapist.com/buyhealthy.php)

Edgy: Mint Double Dark Chocolate Mousse*

Gone wild: Dark chocolate with caramel and tart dried cherries

Cabernet Sauvignon

Grapes used to make: Cabernet sauvignon (at least 75%), merlot, Shiraz

Regions grown in: France/Bordeaux, California (mostly dry cabs), Australia (always dry), Chile, Argentina, Italy, Spain, Washington State

Body: Full-bodied, robust, hearty, big tannins, acidic, deeply colored, concentrated flavors, dense, structured

Flavors: Dark chocolate, black currants, tobacco, blackberry, plum, cherry, mint, green pepper, bitter, woody, vanilla, earth, Havana leaf, espresso, licorice, blueberries, violet, coffee, eucalyptus, spice, truffles, leather, toasty oak

Notes: For centuries, cabernet sauvignon reigned as the world's most planted premium grape, an arguable statement because some sources claim it has been the Grenache grape. Drop back to 2005, and most sites report merlot as number one. There you have it—a continual flux of change. Regardless of its status, the cabernet grape's thick skins make for a bold, tannic, and widely flavorful wine. It's almost the easiest wine to pair with chocolate, second only to tawny port (an opinion, of course).

Adventurous Chocolate Pairings

Conservative: 70% dark chocolate with mint

Edgy: Chocolate chip cookies dipped in melted dark chocolate

Gone wild: Melted 75% dark chocolate with tart dried cherries, chopped pecans, and chopped walnuts; pinch of cinnamon or nutmeg optional

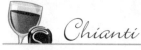 *Chianti*

Grapes used to make: Sangiovese (80%), cabernet sauvignon, merlot, Syrah

Regions grown in: Italy/Tuscany, California/Napa Valley

Body: Light- to medium-bodied, bright acidity, higher in tannins, tannic finish

Flavors: Cherry, bay leaf, coffee, apple, leather, herb, earthy, chocolate, intense dark fruit, citrus in the nose, vanilla, licorice (finish), red plum, cedar, violet, raspberry, toasty oak

Notes: This Italian wine pairs perfectly with Italian entrees like seasoned meats, pizza, sausage, and pasta. This makes it easy to venture out with an Italian-themed dessert such as chocolate tiramisu, a double chocolate hazelnut biscotti, or even a chocolate tortoni.

Adventurous Chocolate Pairings

Conservative: 65% dark single-origin from Madagascar

Edgy: Dark Chocolate Raspberry Meltaway (available by special order at www.TheChocolateTherapist.com)

Gone wild: Chocolate Zabaglione (recipe can be found in *The Little Black Book of Chocolate*)

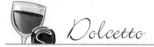 *Dolcetto*

Grapes used to make: Dolcetto

Regions grown in: Italy/Piedmont, Australia, California (where the grapes are called douce noire)

Body: Light- to medium-bodied, easy to drink, low acid

Flavors: Black cherry, licorice, almonds, prunes, fruity, jammy

Notes: "Dolcetto" translates to "little sweet one," but don't look for a little sweet wine here. Although the name implies "wine-cuteness," expect a little tannic snap on the back end from this Italian black grape. Still, it's a lighter wine, so choose a lower-percentage chocolate to avoid overpowering the wine.

Adventurous Chocolate Pairings

Conservative: Chocolate-covered dried Bing cherries

Edgy: Dried cranberries dipped in melted dark chocolate and nutmeg

Gone wild: Dark Chocolate Cake with Chocolate Apricot Glaze,* topped with sliced almonds

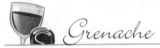

Grenache

Grapes used to make: Grenache

Regions grown in: France, Spain, Italy, California, Australia

Body: Medium- to full-bodied

Flavors: Raisin, currant, spice, blackberry, raspberry, cherry, blueberry, cinnamon, strawberry, vanilla

Notes: Grenache is to France as Garnacha is to Spain—both wines are made from the same grape and work wonderfully with chocolate. Look for a full-bodied selection of this often fruit-forward wine, and choose international brands for excellent quality.

Adventurous Chocolate Pairings

Conservative: Dark chocolate–dipped strawberries

Edgy: Cranberry/Raspberry Chocolate Mousse with Chocolate Whipped Cream (recipe in *The Chocolate Lover's Cookbook for Dummies*)

Gone wild: Wild Women's "Red Hot Mama" all-natural chili pepper truffle (available at www.WildWomenTruffles.com)

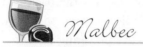 *Malbec*

Grapes used to make: Malbec, occasionally Tannat and cabernet sauvignon

Regions grown in: Argentina, France/Bordeaux

Body: Full, refreshing acidity, sweet tannins

Flavors: Full ripe black fruits, floral tones, leather, vanilla, spice, black raspberry, black cherry, violets, black pepper, anise, smoke, currant, white pepper, boysenberry, sweet toast, licorice, mocha, incense, graphite, mineral

Notes: Most of the wines in Argentina consist of 100 percent of the named grape, which is different from other countries, where you see many blends. Many of the wines are also grown at very high altitudes, with some vineyards as high as ten thousand feet above sea level.

Adventurous Chocolate Pairings

Conservative: Coffee Ganache Truffles*

Edgy: Dark Chocolate Peanut Butter Balls (recipe in *The Chocolate Lover's Cookbook for Dummies*)

Gone wild: Melted dark chocolate with fresh boysenberries, chopped macadamia nuts, and a hint of white pepper

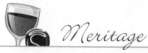 *Meritage*

Grapes used to make: Cabernet sauvignon, merlot, cabernet franc, Petit Verdot, Malbec, Carménère, Gros Verdot. Meritage wines have a required 75% minimum blend of Bordeaux grape varietals.

Regions grown in: California/Napa Valley, Washington, Chile

Body: Medium- to full-bodied with a long finish; can have smooth and soft tannins

Flavors: Dark berries, sweet cherries, spices, coffee, dark cocoa, black olive, floral, plum, toasty oak, berry cobbler, clove, vanilla, blackberry

Notes: The word *Meritage* comes from a combination of the words *merit* and *heritage*, used to describe wines of merit with a superior heritage. For the term to be used on the label, the release must be less than twenty-five thousand bottles and cannot be sold as a bargain-basement wine.

Adventurous Chocolate Pairings

Conservative: Melted milk and dark chocolate swirled with a drop of coffee oil; dipped blackberries optional

Edgy: Dark chocolate with vanilla and chopped pistachios

Gone wild: Melted dark chocolate spiced with ground clove, raisins, and apricot bits

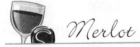 *Merlot*

Grapes used to make: Merlot, cabernet sauvignon

Regions grown in: France/Bordeaux, Italy, Australia, California/Napa Valley, Chile, Argentina, South Africa, New Zealand, Washington State, Long Island

Body: Medium-bodied, soft tannins, supple texture, smooth, rich, easygoing flavor

Flavors: Oak, coffee, black cherry, blackberry, cassis, plum, violet, raisin, vegetable, dark chocolate, coffee, wild blueberry, vanilla, maple syrup, dried herbs, tea, milk chocolate, rose petals, jam

Notes: A broadly versatile wine, merlot spans the food charts in pairing. When venturing into chocolate, think spicy, fruity sauce, walnuts, licorice, and mint, and you'll have a nice start.

Adventurous Chocolate Pairings

Conservative: Dark Chocolate Cherry Truffles*

Edgy: Fresh blackberries in melted dark chocolate with a drop of vanilla

Gone wild: Melted dark chocolate with a drop of black cherry oil and sprinkled with sesame seeds; a dollop of fresh whipping cream sweetened with agave nectar optional

 Mourvèdre

Grapes used to make: Mourvèdre, often blended with Grenache, Syrah, or other Rhône region grapes to improve its color and structure

Regions grown in: Italy, Australia/Barossa Valley, California/Napa Valley, Washington State, Spain, France

Body: Medium- to full-bodied, moderate to full tannins, high in alcohol

Flavors: Cedar, Asian spices, damp earth, game, plum, savory meats, smoky, ripe blackberry, raspberry, black cherry, apricot, chocolate, coffee, leather, oak, tar, toast, sweet wood, herbs

Notes: The savory elements of this grape lend to unlimited pairings, especially with savory chocolate dishes such as Chicken Mole or Jumbo Sea Scallops over Seasoned Cocoa Nibs (www .OpusDine.com). Mourvèdre's unique blend of earthy, gamey, and light red fruit flavors means you shouldn't stop drinking just because dinner has ended—enjoy it with dessert, too!

Adventurous Chocolate Pairings

Conservative: Chocolate and Sea Salt Caramel Tart (recipe in *The Seven Sins of Chocolate*)

Edgy: Dried mango dipped in a melted dark chocolate and ground ginger blend

Gone wild: Poached Apricots with Hot Fudge Sauce (recipe in *The Little Black Book of Chocolate*)

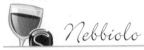

Nebbiolo

Grapes used to make: Nebbiolo

Regions grown in: Italy/Piedmont, California/Napa Valley, Washington, Argentina, Australia

Body: Medium- to full-bodied, silky tannins for a long, fresh finish, although it can be quite tannic when it's younger

Flavors: Roses, ripe fruit, spices, licorice, blackberry, oak, raspberry, cherry, glycerin, coffee, chocolate, smoke, tobacco, berry, plum, tar, herbs, prunes

Notes: This late-harvest grape (October) forms the base of some of Italy's most well-known wines, including Barolo and Barbaresco. It's typically a highly acidic grape, and wines made from the Nebbiolo pair best with the darker chocolates and intensely flavored infusions and inclusions.

Adventurous Chocolate Pairings

Conservative: Organic dried cherries, cinnamon, and dark chocolate

Edgy: Melted dark chocolate with a drop of anise oil and pine nuts

Gone wild: Cranberry Apple Chocolate Chip Crumble (recipe in *I'm Dreaming of a Chocolate Christmas*)

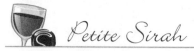

Petite Sirah

Grapes used to make: Petite Sirah, often blended with zinfandel to give it density and structure. The grape is also called Durif.

Regions grown in: California/Napa Valley, Australia, France, Israel

Body: Full-bodied, full tannins, smooth, lasting finish, high acidity, deeply colored

Flavors: Boysenberry, plum, blackberry, black pepper, ink, ripe fruits, jammy, toasty oak, pomegranate, vanilla, dark chocolate, spicy, anise, mocha, smoke

Notes: Like the bold Nebbiolo, this energetic wine is best paired with hearty chocolates and rich, flavorful infusions and inclusions. Its high acidity can easily bury a milder chocolate, so think big—70% dark and higher.

Adventurous Chocolate Pairings

Conservative: Fresh Berry Chocolate Tart (recipe in *The Seven Sins of Chocolate*)

Edgy: Chili Pepper Truffles* (available at www.TheChocolate Therapist.com)

Gone wild: Dark chocolate with cayenne pepper pumpkin seeds (available by special order at www.TheChocolateTherapist .com)

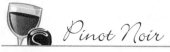

Pinot Noir

Grapes used to make: Pinot noir

Regions grown in: France/Beaujolais, Burgundy, California, Oregon/Willamette Valley, Australia, South Africa, Germany, Switzerland, New Zealand, Italy

Body: Young, light- to medium-bodied, mild to moderate tannin, prominent acidity

Flavors: Cherries, raspberries, earthiness, leather, vanilla, jam, plum, licorice, cedar, mushrooms, strawberries, chocolate, mixed berries, earth, smoke, violet, Asian spices, oak

Notes: A good pinot noir works with practically everything, from potato chips to wild roasted chicken–mushroom risotto. But take note when adding chocolate—give the wine a chance by looking for a medium-bodied, rather than a light-bodied, wine so that you still have a hope of tasting the wine once you've enjoyed your chocolate.

Adventurous Chocolate Pairings

Conservative: Melted milk and dark chocolate, lightly swirled, with fresh blueberries

Edgy: Flourless Chocolate Fantasy (recipe in *The Little Black Book of Chocolate*) drizzled with raspberry puree and sprinkled with finely chopped almonds

Gone wild: Fresh strawberries in melted 50% dark chocolate with a hint of vanilla and Irish Cream; chopped pecans optional

 Port—Ruby

Grapes used to make: Over a hundred grapes can be used in port, but the primary five are Tinta Barroca, Tinta Cao, Tempranillo, Touriga Francesa, and Touriga Nacional.

Regions grown in: Portugal/Douro, Canada, Australia, India, Argentina, South Africa, United States

Body: Full-bodied, fortified (clear brandy is added to port), beautiful deep red colors

Flavors: Dark fruits, red berries, strawberries, raspberries, cherries

Notes: The easiest way to remember which ports pair best with each chocolate is to think about color. Ruby ports pair well with chocolate that has ruby or red-colored fruits like cherries, raspberries, cranberries, strawberries, and pomegranate. Tawny ports (see the next category) work well with tan-colored inclusions, such as nuts, spices, caramel, and toffee.

Adventurous Chocolate Pairings

Conservative: Milk chocolate–covered caramels with sliced strawberries

Edgy: Dried unsweetened mango dipped in melted dark chocolate with cinnamon oil and sprinkled with ground cinnamon

Gone wild: 60% melted dark chocolate with nutmeg, sunflower seeds, and black currants

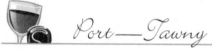

Port—Tawny

Grapes used to make: Over a hundred grapes can be used in port, but the primary five are Tinta Barroca, Tinta Cao, Tempranillo, Touriga Francesa, and Touriga Nacional.

Regions grown in: Portugal/Douro, Canada, Australia, India, Argentina, South Africa, United States

Body: Full-bodied, fortified (clear brandy has been added)

Flavors: Nutty, black pepper, fruit, caramel, toffee, black currant, maple syrup, apricot, orange, date, smoke, spicy, cream

Notes: Tawny port is more delicate and flavorful than ruby port. Just as with the ruby port, the easiest way to remember which ports pair best with each chocolate is to think about color. Tawny ports are tanner in color, so they work best with tan-colored inclusions, such as spices, caramel, toffee, and nuts. Cinnamon is particularly good with tawny port. I highly recommend creating a few of your own cinnamon-infused adventures.

Adventurous Chocolate Pairings

Conservative: Milk chocolate–covered almond toffee (available at www.TheChocolateTherapist.com)

Edgy: Melted 60% dark chocolate with melted caramel and cashews and a pinch of nutmeg

Gone wild: Candied orange peel dipped in lightly swirled, melted dark and milk chocolate with cinnamon oil and sprinkled with hemp seeds

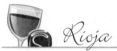 *Rioja*

Grapes used to make: Tempranillo, Garnacha Tinta, Mazuelo, Graciano. True Riojas are composed primarily of Tempranillo (60%) and Garnacha (20%), with the other varietals making up the difference.

Regions grown in: Northern Spain

Body: Medium- to full-bodied, elegant, soft, high alcohol, full and ripe tannins

Flavors: Very fruity, strawberry, oak, vanilla, plum, dark chocolate, cherry, berry, nut, earth, graphite, espresso roast, black currant

Notes: The popular Rioja Gran Reserva wine spends at least two years in an oak barrel and three years in the bottle. Oak and vanilla are the featured flavors, making a vanilla-infused chocolate dessert the perfect partner in pairing.

Adventurous Chocolate Pairings

Conservative: Dark Chocolate Mousse with Bourbon Vanilla Sauce (recipe in *The Chocolate Lover's Cookbook for Dummies*)

Edgy: Black Forest Gateau (recipe in *The Seven Sins of Chocolate*) with Chocolate Whipped Cream*

Gone wild: Melted 75% dark chocolate almonds, macadamia nuts, and dried cherries

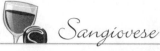

Sangiovese

Grapes used to make: Sangiovese (when cabernet sauvignon, merlot, and Syrah are added, these varietals make up the Super Tuscan wines)

Regions grown in: Italy/Tuscany, California, Argentina, Romania, France, Australia

Body: Light- to medium-bodied, moderate to high acidity

Flavors: Earthy, herbal, black cherry, strawberry, blueberry, floral, plum, violet, orange, clove, cinnamon, thyme

Notes: As Professional Friends of Wine puts it on its Web site, "Sangiovese is to Chianti as Cabernet Sauvignon is to Bordeaux." These grapes form the base of the respective wines, although they can be enjoyable on their own as well. When pairing with chocolate, focus on lighter dark chocolates so that you don't overpower the wine.

Adventurous Chocolate Pairings

Conservative: Fresh strawberries dipped in dark chocolate lightly flavored with cinnamon

Edgy: Chocolate Strawberry Hazelnut Brownie Bars (recipe in *I'm Dreaming of a Chocolate Christmas*)

Gone wild: Melted 55% dark chocolate with a drop of lavender flavoring oil and a dusting of sea salt

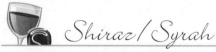

Shiraz / Syrah

Grapes used to make: Shiraz, Viognier, Grenache, Mourvèdre, cabernet sauvignon. Shiraz is almost always blended with other grapes.

Regions grown in: Australia, California, South Africa, France/Rhône Valley. The name Shiraz is primarily used for wines from Australia, South Africa, Argentina, Chile, and Canada, while France and the United States use Syrah. It's the same grape masquerading under separate names.

Body: Full-bodied, generally powerful, robust, long-lived, and tannic

Flavors: Spicy, robust, black pepper, tar, black fruits, plum, blackberries, raspberry, licorice, dark chocolate, bitter chocolate, bitter mocha, floral, cream, rubber, black currants, salt, molasses, caramel, toasty, blueberries, vanilla, acacia flowers, earthy, woody, cola, lychee nuts, blackberry liqueur, cassis, minerality, white chocolate, cinnamon

Notes: A quick review of the many flavors in Shiraz, and it's hard to imagine a chocolate that *doesn't* pair with it. A typically spicy grape, it works nicely with spice-infused chocolates and especially well with eclectic truffles.

Adventurous Chocolate Pairings

Conservative: Dark Chocolate Fondue with cream and raisins; dip desired fruits and nuts into this thick, warm, liquidy chocolate (recipe in *The Seven Sins of Chocolate*)

Edgy: Dark Chocolate Coffee Meltaway drizzled with melted white chocolate (available by special order at www .TheChocolateTherapist.com)

Gone wild: Fresh raspberries dipped in melted dark chocolate swirled with caramel; pinch of black pepper or drop of chili pepper oil optional

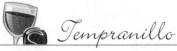 *Tempranillo*

Grapes used to make: This black grape is generally used to make European table wines and port. It's rarely produced as its own wine and, depending on the type of wine being made, will be blended with Grenache, Carignan, Graciano, merlot, and/or cabernet sauvignon.

Regions grown in: Spain, Argentina, South Africa, California/ Napa Valley, Australia, Canada

Body: Medium- to full-bodied, soft, long on finish, low sugar, higher acidity when younger

Flavors: Violet, blackberry, raspberry, truffles, smoke, spices, tobacco, leather, herb, plum, cherry, strawberry, vanilla, oak, and chocolate as it ages

Notes: Like many reds, you can't go wrong with berries and truffles when pairing. Treat it like other full-bodied reds by edging your chocolate toward the darker side.

Adventurous Chocolate Pairings

Conservative: Crème de Menthe Brownie Pie (recipe in *The Little Black Book of Chocolate*)

Edgy: Melted dark chocolate with raisins, nutmeg, and hemp seeds

Gone wild: Gluten-free Hazelnut Biscotti dipped in dark chocolate (recipe in *The Gluten Free Italian Cookbook*)

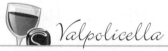

Valpolicella

Grapes used to make: Corvina Veronese, Rondinella, Molinara

Regions grown in: Italy/Veneto, Valpolicella

Body: Light to medium body, full flavor, long finish, fragrant

Flavors: Cherry, raspberry, strawberry, jammy, milk chocolate, licorice, smoky, woodsy, spice, oak, black fruit

Notes: Valpolicella is one of Italy's most produced wines, some say second only to Chianti. Its full fruit flavors and aromas make it easy to pair with chocolate, although consider the lighter darks, as opposed to 70% and higher

Adventurous Chocolate Pairings

Conservative: Melted milk and 50% dark chocolate blend with nutmeg and fresh sliced peaches

Edgy: Licorice and Cinnamon Truffles*

Gone wild: Almond and Coconut Chocolate Chip Tart with Chocolate Merlot Sauce (recipes in *The 300 Best Chocolate Recipes*)

 ## *Zinfandel*

Grapes used to make: Zinfandel, Petite Sirah

Regions grown in: California, Croatia, South Africa, Australia

Body: Generally full-bodied, but can also be medium, usually tannic, rich, big flavor

Flavors: Spicy, smoky, berry, raspberry, blackberry, anise, black cherry, nutty, bitterness, chocolate, pepper, jammy, robust, cinnamon, ginger

Notes: Zinfandel grapes produce a considerably high-alcohol wine, occasionally approaching the 15% alcohol mark. Concerned imbibers will do well with chocolate and nuts, which will help slow absorption of the alcohol into the bloodstream. Spices also work great with this peppy provision.

Adventurous Chocolate Pairings

Conservative: Melted dark chocolate with pistachio nuts, dried cranberries, and sesame seeds

Edgy: Chili Pepper Meltaways (available at www.TheChocolate Therapist.com)

Gone wild: Black Forest Cherry Cake with Raspberry Sauce (recipe in *The Chocolate Lover's Cookbook for Dummies*)

White Wine and Chocolate Pairings

I don't normally pair white wines with chocolate in my classes, but for the sake of research I tossed all preconceived notions aside to create a collection of pairing possibilities for the adventurer. Because there are no precise rules in chocolate and wine pairing, personal discovery is certainly the best measure of success.

White wines are often associated with white grapes, but white wines occasionally include red or even black grapes. The skins are removed prior to fermentation to keep the wine white.

The sweetness of the wine depends on the length of time it's fermented. Wines start out fairly sweet, and as they're allowed to age, the grape's natural sugars are converted into alcohol. Longer processing equates to less sugar, more alcohol, and a drier wine.

More than 90 percent of the world's white wine comes from three grapes—Riesling, sauvignon blanc, and chardonnay. Riesling is considered the sweetest and one of the best to pair with chocolate or a chocolate-based dessert. Sauvignon blanc and chardonnay follow, both of which offer significant pairing challenges as well.

Other white grapes include chenin blanc, Viognier, Sémillon, pinot grigio, pinot blanc, pinot gris, Albarino, and gewürztraminer, but this is far from the entire list. White wine enthusiasts will be thrilled to learn that there are more than fifty major white grape varieties to explore.

As with the red wine discussion, you won't necessarily taste every flavor listed for every wine, but they're included here to help you identify various flavors. Refer to the Wine Aroma Wheel for more ideas.

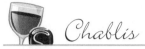

Chablis

Grapes used to make: Chardonnay. Chablis is produced from 100% white grapes, unlike many white wines, which contain a percentage of red grapes as well.

Regions grown in: France/Chablis and Burgundy

Body: Medium- to full-bodied, long finish, dry

Flavors: Lemon, fig, floral, steel, mineral, slate, acidic, crisp, fresh, green apple, soil

Notes: Chablis normally pairs well with cream-based savory dishes, so consider adding a little cream to your chocolate when pairing as well. Because the wine is typically served chilled, let the chocolate dessert sit in your mouth for just a few seconds to begin to melt before you sip the wine.

Adventurous Chocolate Pairings

Conservative: Chocolate Key Lime Pie* with 70% dark melted chocolate

Edgy: Fresh orange wedges dipped in melted dark chocolate and sprinkled with white chocolate shavings

Gone wild: Green apples dipped in a blend of melted caramel and dark chocolate; drop of lemon flavor optional

Champagne

Grapes used to make: Chardonnay, pinot noir, pinot meunier

Regions grown in: France/Champagne (the only authentic Champagne), Italy

Body: White grapes—lighter Champagnes; red grapes—fuller Champagnes; brut/dry, extra dry/semidry, sec/semisweet, demi-sec/sweet

Flavors: Grapefruit, lemon, citrus, apple, yeast, toast, mineral

Notes: Brut and extra dry are better served before and during dinner, while sec and demi-sec work best with chocolate and desserts. Finer Champagnes have smaller bubbles and more of them—look in the narrow part of the Champagne glass to see them best.

Adventurous Chocolate Pairings

Conservative: Fresh strawberries dipped in white chocolate, a Champagne classic

Edgy: Milk chocolate truffles with sea salt

Gone wild: White chocolate rose truffles (available at www .VosgesChocolates.com)

 Chardonnay

Grapes used to make: Chardonnay

Regions grown in: France/Burgundy, California, Australia, Chile, New Zealand, Long Island, Washington State

Body: Typically a dry, medium- to full-bodied wine

Flavors: Tart apple, citrus, lemon, pear, melon, toast, pineapple, vanilla, nuts, butter, wild mushrooms, peach, oak, creamy texture, herb, pear, pineapple, kiwi, smoke, lime zest, jasmine, freesia, honeydew, mineral, earthy, hazelnut

Notes: Chardonnay is generally aged in oak barrels and has a rich, buttery flavor. This makes it an obvious choice for luscious apple pie and chocolate, among other chocolate delights.

Adventurous Chocolate Pairings

Conservative: Thinly sliced tart green apples dipped in milk chocolate with an optional light sprinkling of sea salt

Edgy: Chocolate Apple Cobbler (recipe in *The Seven Sins of Chocolate*)

Gone wild: Key Lime Pie with Raspberry Chocolate Sauce (recipe in *The Chocolate Lover's Cookbook for Dummies*)

 Chenin Blanc

Grapes used to make: Chenin blanc

Regions grown in: California, France/Loire Valley, South Africa, Australia

Body: Crisp, dry wine with high acidity; ranges from very dry to very sweet, depending on the region where it's grown. Light to medium body, occasionally made as dessert wine.

Flavors: Apple pie, pear, tart green apple, floral, honey, nuttiness, wax, damp straw, honeycomb, pepper, grapes, apricots, fruit flowers, mineral, melon, lime, nectarine, peach, quince, cloves, cream

Notes: Chenin blanc offers up a bit of challenge for chocolate pairing, with its high acidity, so be prepared for true adventure!

Adventurous Chocolate Pairings

Conservative: Tart apple pie drizzled with melted 70% dark chocolate and sprinkled with nutmeg

Edgy: Dried peaches dipped in 55% dark chocolate blended with a drop of clove oil (or with powdered clove sprinkled on)

Gone wild: Whole pecans dipped in melted dark chocolate blended with a drop of lemon oil; shake of chili pepper optional

Gewürztraminer

Grapes used to make: Gewürztraminer

Regions grown in: France/Alsace, California, Germany, Northern Italy, Washington State, Austria

Body: Medium-bodied, lower acidity, spicy, low-alcohol, ranges from sweet to dry depending on where the grapes are grown and the time they're harvested

Flavors: Allspice, clove, floral, cinnamon, ginger, white pepper, rose water, lychee nut, citrus, honeysuckle, pink grapefruit, green apple, melon, apricot, peach, mint, licorice, roasted almond, high fruity flavors

Notes: Depending on how it's produced, this highly fruit-flavored wine is often quite sweet. Look for a late-harvest Gerwürztraminer for added sweetness. As such, it lends itself nicely to a variety of chocolate pairings. Keep fruit in the picture for best results.

Adventurous Chocolate Pairings

Conservative: Chocolate Candied Orange Strips (recipes in *Chocolat*)

Edgy: Ginger cookies dipped in Pear Jam and Chocolate (recipe in *The Seven Sins of Chocolate*)

Gone wild: Chocolate Truffle Tort with Raspberry Sauce (recipe *in The Chocolate Lover's Cookbook for Dummies*)

Muscat / Moscato

Grapes used to make: Muscat (considered the oldest varietal of all grapes)

Regions grown in: France/Loire Valley, Greece, Italy/Piedmont, Australia, California, Chile

Body: Generally a lighter, sweet, low-alcohol wine, very often a bit bubbly. Wines from Alsace tend to be drier. Head to southern France for sweet dessert wines.

Flavors: Peach, apricot, orange, honey, floral, spice, berry, tangerine, lemon, grape, musky, pear, white flowers. Flavors vary, depending on the region—Alsace and Samos have more tangerine, while Moscato d'Asti is more of a honey and floral wine.

Notes: The muscat grape is considered the oldest varietal of all grapes. This very sweet, low-alcohol dessert wine pairs wonderfully with orange fruits—oranges, apricots, peaches, mangos, papayas—and milk or dark chocolate, or both . . . why not?

Adventurous Chocolate Pairings

Conservative: Dried mango dipped in a melted milk/dark chocolate blend; sprinkling of cinnamon optional

Edgy: Fresh orange and peach slices with Chocolate Whipped Cream*

Gone wild: Chopped figs, chopped pecans, and chopped apricot bits, all tossed in melted 55% dark chocolate

 Pinot Blanc

Grapes used to make: Pinot blanc

Regions grown in: Oregon, California, Italy/Alto Adige, France/Alsace

Body: High acid, low sugar, clean, dry and crisp, long finish, typically light to medium body

Flavors: Melons, peaches, nectar, honey, mineral, lime zest, nectarine, vanilla, wet stones, cider, chalk, lemon zest, walnut, green apple, spice

Notes: This clean, crisp wine makes a nice opening cocktail, guaranteed to wake up your guests and bring everyone into the moment. Once all of you are there, make sure they stay focused with an array of spicy, fruit-chocolate options.

Adventurous Chocolate Pairings

Conservative: Melted dark chocolate with cinnamon and roasted and salted macadamia nuts

Edgy: Thinly sliced red apples topped with Havarti cheese and melted 45% dark chocolate

Gone wild: Blue cheese crumbles, walnuts, and honey mixed together, drizzled with 55% dark chocolate; sprinkling of nutmeg optional

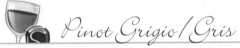

Pinot Grigio / Gris

Grapes used to make: Pinot grigio or pinot gris

Regions grown in: France/Alsace, Italy, California, Oregon, New Zealand, Austria

Body: Sometimes dry and spicy, sometimes sweet. A special wine for those who simply can't (or won't) make up their minds. Typically full-bodied and sweet.

Flavors: Spice, honey, nutty, fruity, smoke, pastry

Notes: Flavors vary considerably from region to region, but chances are good you'll be happy with high-acidity fruits that match the acidity of the wine. Dare you go where no man has paired before?

Adventurous Chocolate Pairings

Conservative: Melted dark chocolate over fresh pineapple wedges sprinkled with chopped almonds

Edgy: Lemon meringue pie drizzled with melted 50% dark chocolate

Gone wild: Double Chocolate Biscotti (recipe in *The Chocolate Lover's Cookbook for Dummies*) dipped in melted dark chocolate with pistachio nuts and dried cranberries

 *Riesling*

Grapes used to make: Riesling

Regions grown in: Germany, Australia, France/Alsace, Washington State, New York, Austria, California/Sonoma, New Zealand, Italy, Canada, China, Italy

Body: Light-bodied, crisp and sharp acidity, low alcohol. Depending on the region, can be dry, semisweet, sweet, or sparkling.

Flavors: Honey, floral, apple, pear, peach, melon, minerals, petrol, kerosene, rubber, mango, guava, citrus notes, vanilla, apricot, orange, lime, slate, strawberry cream, lychee

Notes: Select a late-harvest Riesling when pairing with chocolate—you'll get a sweeter wine better suited to chocolate desserts.

Adventurous Chocolate Pairings

Conservative: Dried peach dipped in melted dark chocolate sweetened with ½ teaspoon of agave nectar and chopped strawberries

Edgy: Chocolate Mandarin Truffle Cake (recipe in *I'm Dreaming of a Chocolate Christmas*)

Gone wild: Thinly sliced dark chocolate, Brie cheese, and crushed filberts

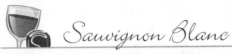

Sauvignon Blanc

Grapes used to make: Sauvignon blanc, Sémillon

Regions grown in: France, California, Australia, Chile, South Africa, Washington State, New Zealand

Body: Medium- to full-bodied, depending on the maker; generally high acidity, crisp, clear; dryer wines come from Graves and Pessac-Léognan, while the sweeter options hail from Sauternes and Barsac.

Flavors: Grapefruit, zesty, gooseberry, asparagus, fruit salad, smoky, haylike, tangy, fresh herbs, lime, citrus, mineral, lemongrass, plum, straw, passion fruit, kiwi, pear, cantaloupe, orange peel, cut grass

Notes: Also known as fumé blanc; expect a grassy flavor and possibly some oak, along with its typically acidic fruit flavors. Definitely a long shot when pairing with chocolate but guaranteed excitement for the true adventurer.

Adventurous Chocolate Pairings

Conservative: Kiwi dipped in melted milk chocolate infused with ground nutmeg

Edgy: Grapefruit wedges topped with 45% melted dark chocolate, sprinkled with sesame seeds

Gone wild: Chocolate Valencia Pie (recipe in *The Colorado Colore*), drizzled with melted dark chocolate and optional Chocolate Whipped Cream*

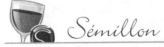

Sémillon

Grapes used to make: Sémillon, sauvignon blanc, Muscadelle, Chardonnay

Regions grown in: France/Bordeaux, Australia, California, Washington, Chile

Body: Light- to medium-bodied, low acidity

Flavors: Lime, toast, cheese, peach, apricot, herb, honey, citrus, pineapple, vanilla

Notes: Sémillon is more often blended with other grapes, rather than offered on its own. Dry wine enthusiasts will want to choose wines from the Sauternes region of Bordeaux. Those looking for sweeter fare would do well with Australian and Washington wines.

Adventurous Chocolate Pairings

Conservative: Dried apricot halves dipped in melted dark chocolate

Edgy: Thin rice crackers topped with melted Havarti cheese and dark chocolate shavings

Gone wild: Fresh pineapple dipped in melted dark chocolate with cinnamon and raw sunflower seeds

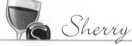

Sherry

Grapes used to make: Palomino, Pedro Ximénez

Regions grown in: Spain, Germany, Italy, France

Body: Dry/manzanilla; dry/fino; dry to medium-dry/amontillado; dry to medium-dry/oloroso; sweet/cream

Flavors: Nutty, caramel, hazelnuts, walnut, fig, molasses, dates, smoky, green apple

Notes: Sherry is a fortified wine, meaning neutral brandy has been added to the wine to raise the alcohol content. With sherry, the brandy is added after fermentation. In port, it's added before. Cream sherry pairs wonderfully with chocolate, but don't hesitate to venture into a little of everything.

Adventurous Chocolate Pairings

> **Conservative:** Figs dipped in milk chocolate
>
> **Edgy:** Dark chocolate with currants and chopped walnuts
>
> **Gone wild:** Double Dark Chocolate Brownies* topped with melted chocolate and caramel and chopped almonds

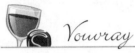

Vouvray

Grapes used to make: Chenin blanc

Regions grown in: France

Body: Dry, semisweet, or sweet

Flavors: Fruit, mineral, lemon, apple, pear, peach, floral

Notes: Now is as good a time as any to pull out this much-loved cliché: "Life is like a box of chocolates . . . you never know what you're going to get"—unless, of course, you know your Vouvrays. The wine varies greatly from region to region, like so many of our friendly whites. Sweeter is generally better with chocolates.

Adventurous Chocolate Pairings

> **Conservative:** Red apple slices with melted Monterey Jack cheese and topped with semisweet dark chocolate chips
>
> **Edgy:** Chocolate Peach Cobbler* sprinkled with chopped cashews; melted chocolate on top optional
>
> **Gone wild:** Chocolate Fruity Cakes (recipe in *I'm Dreaming of a Chocolate Christmas*) topped with dark chocolate sauce and pine nuts

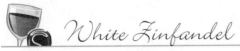

White Zinfandel

Grapes used to make: Zinfandel

Regions grown in: California

Body: Light, soft, low in alcohol, sweet

Flavors: Vanilla, cherry, orange, raspberry, lime, plum, tangy, strawberry, pineapple, pear

Notes: White zinfandel is made from red zinfandel grapes that have had the skins peeled off before fermentation. The resulting wine is very light, generally quite sweet, and often snubbed by true wine enthusiasts. Fabulous! This means more for those who appreciate a relaxed, fresh wine that offers a collection of interesting chocolate pairings.

Adventurous Chocolate Pairings

Conservative: Sliced pears dipped into melted milk chocolate with coconut flakes

Edgy: Melted 50% dark chocolate with dried blueberries, roasted and salted sunflower seeds, and a pinch of nutmeg

Gone wild: Chocolate Orange Breton Sable (recipe in *The Seven Sins of Chocolate*)

Reference Guide

For your dining and wining pleasure, here is a quick of list of what fruits, nuts, and other treats go best with what wine.

Moscato	Pinot Noir	Zinfandel	Cabernet
Peach	Blueberries	Cinnamon	Cherries
Mango	Cashews	Pecans	Raspberries
Apricot	Milk chocolate	Nutmeg	Almonds
Orange	Blackberries	Chile pepper	Blackberries
Nectarine	Hemp seeds	Strawberries	Mint

Wine Shopping Ideas

You can either pair the wine with the chocolate or the chocolate with the wine. I generally start with the chocolate and pair it with the wine because I like chocolate more than wine. For me, having the perfect chocolate outweighs the importance of the wine. Many people, however, prefer to choose the wine first and pair the chocolate with the wine.

Smaller specialty shops generally offer wines that the owners or the buyers have tasted and hand-selected. For diversity, look for stores with a nice international selection that includes wines from Argentina, Chile, South Africa, New Zealand, and Australia.

If you already have your chocolate or dessert idea in mind, look for wines that list similar flavors to what you're serving. Many wines have entertaining and informative descriptions on the labels, but if not, this is where the store owner or the information cards above the wines (in some stores) will come in handy.

Chocolate and Wine Pairing Guidelines

- Taste both the chocolate and the wine in the same order, as if you were at an individual chocolate-tasting or wine-tasting event. Sample lighter wines and chocolates first, and move to darker from there.

- Eat salt-free crackers or pretzels and drink a little water between pairings to cleanse your palate.

- It's best to taste no more than six wines and chocolates in a single event. After that, taste buds can become desensitized and lose their ability to differentiate flavors.

- Typically, light wines work better with a lighter chocolate, while the heavier, more robust wines need darker chocolates. A heavy wine can overpower the chocolate, and vice versa.

- Fortified wines (i.e., port, sherry) pair exceptionally well with chocolate because they're sweeter, and the wine's structure pairs well with chocolate.

- Wines with similar attributes as the chocolate work well together. For example, a fruity wine will better serve a chocolate with fruit nuances. This is called synergy—the two ideally match each other in some way and enhance the flavors of both.

- A sweeter chocolate, such as milk or white chocolate, can make some wines taste bitter and astringent. Again, work to match the sweetness of the wine to the sweetness of the chocolate.

- Bittersweet chocolates generally go best with stronger red wines, especially wines that may have a slightly roasted and bitter flavor with their own chocolate notes.

- Milk and white chocolates pair well with dessert wines such as moscato, port, and very sweet white wines.

- Tannic wines work wonderfully with rich, heavy chocolates that have extra cocoa butter or cream. The butter in the chocolate helps mellow the tannic element of the wine.

- Remember port pairings by their colors—ruby port pairs well with ruby-colored infusions like berries, cherries, and strawberries. Tawny port generally works quite well with tawny (or tan) colored infusions, such as nuts, caramel, spices, and toffees.

Wine Information Web Sites

Bon Appétit	www.epicurious.com
Decanter	www.decanter.com
Easy French Food	www.EasyFrenchFood.com
Food and Wine	www.FoodandWine.com
Gourmet Sleuth	www.GourmetSleuth.com
Happy Hour Alert	www.HappyHourAlert.com
My Wines Direct	www.MyWinesDirect.com
Professional Friends of Wine	www.WinePros.com
Wine and Spirits	www.wineandspiritsmagazine.com
Wine Club Central	www.WineClubCentral.com
Wine Enthusiast	www.WineMag.com
Wine Intro	www.WineIntro.com
Wine Making	www.WineMaking.com
Wine Spectator	www.WineSpectator.com
Wine.com	www.Wine.com

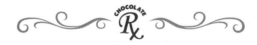

Nine

Recipes

*I*F YOU HAVE AN ORIGINAL chocolate recipe that you'd like to see featured in my next book, please e-mail it to julie@thechocolatetherapist.com.

Include your full name and a note with your permission to reprint the recipe.

How to Microwave Chocolate

Many of the suggested wine and chocolate pairings call for you to make your own concoctions of melted chocolate, nuts, berries, spices, and/or naturally flavored oils. This quick section will have you creating your own extraordinary recipes in no time. In 1½ to 3 minutes, your chocolate creation will be ready to go.

Chocolate is a bit finicky. When heated improperly, your delightful dish can turn into a scorched, "seized" chocolate mass. Fortunately, once you learn the technique, it's almost fail-proof.

The main caveats in microwaving chocolate are to do it slowly and to use low heat. It also works best in a glass bowl (not ceramic or plastic). Make sure there's absolutely no water in the bowl, or your chocolate may seize up into an ugly chunk.

1. Pour the chocolate into the bowl until it's about half full.
2. Reduce the microwave heat to 50 percent.
3. Microwave for 30 seconds, remove the bowl, and stir the chocolate (not much has happened yet).
4. Reduce the heat 50 percent again.
5. Microwave it again for 30 seconds, remove, and stir.
6. Let the chocolate begin to melt on its own.
7. Reduce the heat to 50 percent, microwave, and stir again.
8. Repeat as needed, always remembering to reduce the heat each time.

Remove the chocolate just before it is completely melted, and stir the remaining chunks until they melt. Melted chocolate is best for dipping, mixing, and serving immediately. It won't naturally harden into the same form it was in before you started unless you've "tempered" it, or brought it up and down to the exact heat required to reset the original form. If you want to dip chocolates that you plan to serve later, you'll need to refrigerate them to get them to harden.

Tempering is best done with a tempering machine—I've tried doing it in the microwave and on the stove with a candy thermometer, and it works great if you happen to have an extra ten days to experiment. Short of that, use the refrigerator or buy a tempering machine.

Chocolate Kahlúa Truffles

KRISTIN RENZEMA

12 ounces semisweet dark chocolate chips
½ cup heavy cream (*not* half-and-half)
½ stick butter (do not use margarine)
1 tablespoon instant coffee granules
2 tablespoons Kahlúa
¼ teaspoon salt
Cocoa powder for dusting

Combine all of the ingredients except the cocoa powder in a small saucepan. Heat over low heat, stirring occasionally, until very smooth. Chill the mixture, covered, in the refrigerator until it's firm (approximately 1 hour). Take heaping tablespoons of the mixture, form them into 1-inch balls, and roll each ball in the cocoa powder. Store the truffles in the refrigerator or the freezer for up to 1 month.

Chocolate Drop Cookies

LIANNE MCCRIRICK

2 cups brown sugar
1 cup butter

2 eggs, beaten
4 squares organic dark baking chocolate, melted
1 cup milk
4 cups flour
1 teaspoon baking soda
½ cup chopped walnuts
Dark cocoa powder (optional)
Powdered sugar (optional)

Preheat the oven to 350 degrees Fahrenheit.

In a medium bowl, cream the sugar and butter, add the eggs and chocolate, then add the milk. Blend together well. Sift together the flour and baking soda, add to the chocolate mixture, and stir. Add the walnuts and stir until well combined. Drop spoonfuls of the batter onto a greased baking sheet and bake for approximately 10 minutes.

Dust the cookies lightly with a mixture of dark cocoa powder and powdered sugar after baking, if desired.

Chocolate Key Lime Pie

This is a speed baker's no-bake version.

1 can (14 ounces) sweetened condensed milk
Juice from 2 lemons
Juice from 4 limes
1½ cups heavy whipping cream (or use 16 ounces Cool Whip)
¼ cup baking cocoa powder
4 tablespoons pure cane sugar or agave nectar
1 prepared graham cracker crust

In a small bowl, mix the milk with the juice of the lemons and limes and set aside. In a medium bowl, blend the heavy cream with a blender until it forms stiff peaks. Stir in the cocoa powder and sugar, then add the juice-milk mixture. Stir until just mixed.

Pour the mixture into the prepared crust and refrigerate for at least 1 hour before serving.

Chocolate Mug Cake

ROSE SIMONELLI

4 tablespoons flour (for a gluten-free version, use oat flour)
4 tablespoons sugar or agave nectar
2 tablespoons baking cocoa powder
Pinch of salt
1 egg
3 tablespoons milk (or almond milk)
3 tablespoons coconut oil
2 drops pure vanilla extract
3 tablespoons dark chocolate chips
3 tablespoons walnuts or pecans (optional)

Mix the flour, sugar, cocoa powder, and salt together in a large glass coffee mug. Add the egg and mix it into the dry ingredients. Add the rest of the ingredients and mix thoroughly. Bake in the microwave on high for 3 minutes.

Chocolate Peach Cobbler

¼ cup organic brown sugar
4 teaspoons cornstarch
¾ cup water
½ teaspoon pure vanilla extract
½ teaspoon cinnamon or nutmeg
5 cups fresh sliced peaches
¼ cup (½ stick) butter
1 cup flour
1 teaspoon baking powder

1 egg
¼ cup milk
1 tablespoon agave nectar
1 cup (or more) dark chocolate chips

Preheat the oven to 400 degrees Fahrenheit.

Combine the brown sugar, cornstarch, water, vanilla, and spices in a large saucepan, bring to a boil, and then simmer until the mixture is thickened, approximately 15 minutes. Add the peaches and 1 tablespoon of the butter and heat through; remove from the heat and set aside.

To make the biscuitlike crust, mix the flour and baking powder in a large bowl, then cut in the rest of the butter until the flour is crumbly. Blend the egg and milk and add along with the agave nectar to the flour mixture; stir until doughy. Add a little extra milk if the dough is too tacky. Spoon the peaches into a 9 × 12-inch pan and sprinkle 1 cup (or more, if you prefer) of dark chocolate chips over the peaches. Top them with the biscuit dough mixture—either sprinkle it randomly across the peaches or roll it into 8 to 10 round biscuits and arrange them on top to form individual servings. Bake the cobbler for 20 minutes.

Chocolate Whipped Cream

½ cup heavy cream
1 tablespoon cocoa powder
1 tablespoon pure cane sugar or ½ tablespoon agave nectar
Grated dark chocolate (optional)

In a medium bowl, whip the cream with a handheld mixer until it forms stiff peaks. Add the cocoa powder and sugar (adjust to your taste) and blend in.

To really impress guests, sprinkle some grated dark chocolate on top of the whipped cream.

Dark Chocolate Cake with Chocolate/Apricot Glaze

This is a speed baker's version, using a box of chocolate cake mix.

1 box chocolate cake mix, any brand
¼ cup baking cocoa powder

While preparing the cake according to the package directions, add the baking cocoa powder to the batter. Bake the cake and set aside to cool.

Chocolate/Apricot Glaze

1 cup pure apricot preserves (no sugar added)
½ cup orange juice
1 tablespoon agave nectar or honey
½ cup dark chocolate chips or chopped dark chocolate bar

In a small saucepan, combine the preserves, orange juice, and agave nectar and stir over medium heat until melted. Reduce the heat to low and stir in the chocolate chips. Simmer uncovered on low heat for 15 minutes, or until the mixture is thick enough to stay on the back of a spoon. Drizzle or brush the glaze over the cake.

Dark Vanilla Chocolate Drizzle

8 ounces dark chocolate chips
1 teaspoon pure vanilla extract (do not use vanillin, an artificial flavoring)

Put the chocolate chips in a glass bowl. Microwave them on low heat, 30 seconds at a time, stirring each time, until the chocolate is melted. Add the vanilla and stir. Drizzle onto a pie or anything else!

Double Dark Chocolate Brownies

This is a speed baker's rendition, using a boxed brownie mix.

1 box brownie mix, any brand

Add to the mixture
¼ cup baking cocoa, preferably undutched
1 cup dark chocolate chips or one 3-ounce dark chocolate bar, chopped

Preheat the oven to the temperature specified in the brownie mix directions.

Follow the rest of the directions on the brownie box. Add the cocoa and chocolate chips to the batter and bake the brownies according to the directions on the box.

Gluten-Free Chocolate/Chocolate-Chip Oatmeal Cookies

This is my own special invention, developed out of necessity for my gluten-intolerant son. You'll never believe these are gluten-free!

½ cup shortening
¼ cup butter
¾ cup organic brown sugar
2 teaspoons pure vanilla extract
3 eggs

2 ½ cups oat flour (make your own by grinding old-fashioned
   oats in the blender)
¼ cup organic dark cocoa powder
1 teaspoon salt
1 teaspoon baking soda
3 cups regular oats (not quick-cooking)
2 3.5-ounce organic dark chocolate bars, chopped
¾ cup pecans, chopped (optional)

Preheat the oven to 340 degrees Fahrenheit.

In a large bowl, combine the shortening, butter, brown
sugar, and vanilla and stir by hand until blended. (I prefer to stir
cookie mix by hand because the cookies come out thicker and
chewier than if you use an electric mixer. But feel free to choose
either method.) Add the eggs and stir well. Add the flour, cocoa
powder, salt, and baking soda and mix well. Stir in the oats and
mix. Add the chopped chocolate and pecans (if using) and stir
to distribute them throughout the mixture.

Drop tablespoonfuls of the batter onto a lightly greased
cookie sheet and bake for 9 to 10 minutes.

Haute Chocolate

**To make this recipe lighter, substitute vanilla almond milk or
rice milk, but note that the mixture will not get as thick as
when you use half-and-half or whole milk. Also, you may
want to try this without a sweetener, as the half-and-half
makes the chocolate much sweeter.**

4 ounces 65%+ dark chocolate, chocolate chips, or a chocolate bar
2½ cups half-and-half or whole milk
3 tablespoons undutched cocoa powder
½ teaspoon pure vanilla extract
2 tablespoons agave nectar or other sweetener (optional)
¼ teaspoon ancho or cayenne chili powder (optional)
Whipped cream and chopped nuts (optional)

Chop the chocolate into very fine pieces.

Pour the half-and-half into a medium saucepan and turn the heat to medium, stirring constantly.

Turn the heat to low, whisk in the chocolate and cocoa powder, and allow to simmer until the liquid has thickened slightly (make sure it doesn't boil).

Add the vanilla, agave nectar, and ancho (if using), stir, then pour the liquid into 4 small coffee or tea cups. Garnish each cup with whipped cream and chopped nuts, if you prefer, and serve.

Super Fast Hot Chocolate

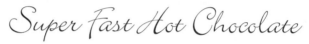

1 cup milk (rice, soy, almond and coconut milk can be substituted for a dairy-free treat)
1½ teaspoons sugar or sugar substitute
2 teaspoons Rapunzel 100% organic cocoa powder (or brand of your choice)
1 drop pure vanilla extract
Dash of cinnamon (optional)

Mix all of the ingredients together in a mug and microwave for 1 minute, 40 seconds. Alternatively, mix the ingredients together in a small pan and heat them slowly on the stove, stirring constantly, until the desired temperature is reached, about 3 minutes.

Mint Double Dark Chocolate Mousse

DEETTE KOZLOW

6 ounces organic extra dark chocolate
3 tablespoons Grand Marnier

5 large eggs, separated
3 tablespoons sugar
1¼ cups milk
½ teaspoon peppermint oil

Chop the chocolate into small pieces and combine it with the Grand Marnier in the top part of a double boiler. Heat slowly until the chocolate is melted.

In a medium bowl, whisk the egg yolks and 2 tablespoons of the sugar until the yolks are light and airy in texture; set aside.

In a medium saucepan, heat the milk until it's not quite boiling. Remove from the heat and add the egg yolk and sugar mixture, stirring constantly. Return the pan to medium heat and stir until the milk mixture thickens enough to coat the back of a spoon, approximately 15 minutes.

Add the melted chocolate and Grand Marnier to the egg yolk, sugar, and milk mixture and stir until well blended. Remove from the heat and set aside.

In another medium bowl, beat the egg whites until they're foamy. Add the remaining tablespoon of sugar and continue beating until the egg whites are stiff. Carefully fold them into the chocolate mixture. Stir in the peppermint oil and mix well. Pour the mousse into 6 to 8 dessert cups, chill them for several hours, and serve.

Pomegranate and Cinnamon Double Dark Chocolate Brownies

Use the Double Dark Chocolate Brownies recipe (see page 224), but when making the brownie mix, substitute pomegranate juice for the water in the recipe and add 1 teaspoon of cinnamon to the batter.

Raspberry / Pomegranate Puree

1 pound frozen raspberries, thawed and drained
½ cup plus 2 tablespoons pomegranate juice
⅓ cup agave nectar, honey, or raw cane sugar
1 tablespoon cornstarch

Combine the raspberries, ½ cup of the pomegranate juice, and your sweetener of choice in a medium saucepan and bring to a boil; then allow it to simmer for 15 minutes. Dissolve the cornstarch in the remaining 2 tablespoons of the pomegranate juice and add this to the simmering mixture, stirring constantly. Continue to simmer until the puree is thickened. Spoon the puree over brownies, chocolate cake, chocolate pies, or the dessert of your choice.

Raspberry Truffle Brownies

KRISTIN RENZEMA

¾ cup (1½ sticks) butter
4 ounces organic unsweetened dark chocolate, chopped
3 large eggs
2 cups sugar
⅓ cup raspberry jam
3 tablespoons black raspberry liqueur
1 cup all-purpose flour
¼ teaspoon salt
1 cup dark chocolate chips
Powdered sugar (optional)

Preheat the oven to 350 degrees Fahrenheit.

Spray a 9-inch-diameter springform pan with nonstick cooking spray. Melt the butter and chocolate in a large saucepan over low heat, stirring constantly until smooth. Remove from the heat and set aside. Whisk in the eggs, sugar, jam, and liqueur. Stir in the flour and salt, then the chocolate chips. Transfer the batter to the prepared pan.

Bake the truffle brownies until a toothpick inserted in the center comes out with moist crumbs attached, about 45 minutes. Let them cool in the pan on a rack for about an hour. When the brownies have cooled completely, run a small knife around the edges of the pan to help loosen them, then cut them into 12 squares. Dust the brownies with powdered sugar, if you prefer.

Tart Apple/Blackberry Pie

3 pounds thinly sliced green apples
1 pound fresh or frozen (thawed and drained) blackberries
¼ cup lemon juice
¾ cup pure cane sugar or raw sugar
½ cup flour (or ¾ cup oat flour for less gluten)
1 teaspoon powdered cinnamon
½ teaspoon powdered cloves
Butter (softened)
Frozen pastry crust for single-crust pie, thawed and ready for
   baking

Preheat the oven to 375 degrees Fahrenheit.

In a large bowl, combine the apples, blackberries, and lemon juice and stir to coat the fruit with the lemon juice. In a small bowl, combine the sugar, flour, cinnamon, and cloves until blended. Add the dry mixture to the apples and blackberries and toss until the fruit is well coated. Lightly butter the bottom of the pie crust. Pour the mixture into the pie crust and cover with foil. Bake the pie for 30 minutes. Remove the foil and bake for another 30 minutes, or until the apples are slightly soft (test lightly with a fork).

Truffles

8 ounces whipping cream
½ cup (1 stick) butter
16 ounces 60%+ dark chocolate, melted
Oils (see below)
Pure cocoa powder, or cocoa powder and powdered-sugar mixture

In a medium saucepan, heat the whipping cream over medium heat until it's boiling, stirring constantly. Remove from the heat, add the butter, and continue stirring until it's melted. Slowly add the butter and cream mixture to the melted chocolate. Add the various oils listed below, depending on the recipe.

Allow the truffle mixture to sit uncovered until it reaches room temperature, stirring occasionally. To speed up the process, the mixture can be put in the refrigerator until it reaches a consistency that can be rolled. Roll spoonfuls into ½-inch balls, then roll each ball in pure cocoa powder, a cocoa powder and powdered-sugar mixture, or various spices. The truffles can also be dipped in melted chocolate and refrigerated.

Add more flavors, if desired—the following recommendations are starting points. Note that if you have extra-strong flavoring oils, you may need less than these listed amounts. Start with small amounts and add a little at a time to flavor the truffles.

The flavors listed here are oils, not flavorings or extracts. Oils are much stronger and are designed to flavor chocolates, so make sure you're using oils and not water-based extracts. You may purchase organic chocolate-flavoring oils at www.NaturesFlavors .com.

Chili Pepper Truffles: ½ tablespoon chili oil
Coffee Ganache Truffles: ½ tablespoon coffee oil
Dark Chocolate Cherry Truffles: ½ tablespoon cherry oil

Licorice and Cinnamon Truffles: ¼ tablespoon anise oil,
  ¼ tablespoon cinnamon oil
Licorice Raspberry Truffles: ¼ tablespoon raspberry oil,
  ¼ tablespoon anise oil
Raspberry Dark Chocolate Truffles: ½ tablespoon
  raspberry oil

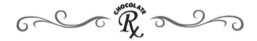

Appendix A

The Chocolate Bible

Everything You Need to Survive

Here you'll find Web sites, brands by country, research, and other must-have chocolate information.

Worldwide Shopping

Bella Cabosse: Artisan chocolates
   from around the world
www.bellacabosse.com

Belgian Chocolate Online
www.chocolat.com

Chocolate by Sparrow: International
   chocolate collection
www.chocolatebysparrow.com

Chocolate 4 U: International
   chocolate company
www.chocolate4u.com

Chocolate Gelt: Largest selection of
   chocolate gelt online
www.chocolategelt.com

The Chocolate Life: "Chocophiles"
   informational Web site
www.thechocolatelife.com

The Chocolate Path: The best
   everyday dark chocolate
www.chocolatepath.com

Chocolate of the Month Club
www.chocolatemonthclub.com

Chocolate Therapist: All-natural
   milk and dark chocolate with
   natural infusions and inclusions
www.TheChocolateTherapist.com

Chocolate Trading Company: A
   wide selection of chocolate from
   around the world
www.chocolatetradingcompany.com

Chocosphere: International chocolate collection
www.chocosphere.com

Fine Dark Chocolate: Products from and information about high-quality chocolate companies
www.finedarkchocolate.com

Global Chocolates: Corporate, retail, and wholesale European chocolates
www.globalchocolates.com

Mostly Chocolate: Fine premium chocolates and more
www.mostlychocolate.com

Vermont Nutfree Chocolates: Completely nut-free chocolates
www.VermontNutfree.com

World Wide Chocolate: Gourmet chocolates from around the world
www.worldwidechocolate.com

ZChocolate: Worldwide chocolate, international express delivery
www.zchocolate.com

International Brands by Country

Belgium
Café Tasse: www.cafe-tasse.com

Callebaut: Belgian chocolate, retail throughout the world; also a supplier for chocolate makers
www.barry-callebaut.com

Cavalier: No sugar-added chocolate
www.cavalier.be

Chocoa: All-natural Belgian chocolate
www.chocoa.com

Côte d'Or
www.cotedor.be

Dolfin
www.chocosphere.com

Galler
www.galler.com

Neuhaus: Unique Belgian chocolates
www.neuhaus-online-store.com

New Tree
www.newtree.com

Nirvana: Exquisite, handcrafted Belgian chocolates
www.nirvanachocolates.com

Colombia
Santander: Quality chocolate since 1920
www.chocolates.com

Ecuador
Pacari: Single-origin, organic, raw, and Fair Trade chocolate bars
www.pacarichocolate.com

Plantations
Purchase at www.worldwidechocolate.com

Republica del Cacao: Single-origin bars made from the rare and exquisite Arriba bean
www.republicadelcacao.com

France
Bernard Castelain
Purchase at www.worldwidechocolate.com or www.chocosphere.com

Bonnat: Chocolates and confections since 1884
www.bonnat-chocolatier.com

Chocolaterie Weiss: More than 125 years of French chocolate-making perfection poured into every product
www.chocolate-weiss.com

L'Ancienne: Delightful French drinking chocolate, powdered cocoa
Purchase at www.chocosphere.com

Jean-Paul Hévin: Chocolate for the refined chocolate aficionado
www.jphevin.com

Marquise de Sévigné: Mouthwatering traditional manufacturing–style French chocolates since 1892
www.marquise-de-sevigne.com

Michel Cluizel: Founded in 1948, Michel Cluizel sets its focus on the quality and uniqueness of the cocoa beans selected for production
www.cluizel.com

Pralus: Luxury French chocolate made from the finest beans available
www.chocolats-pralus.com
Purchase at www.chocosphere.com

Richart: Beautifully boxed, exceptional culinary combinations
www.richart-chocolates.com

Valrhona: Founded in 1922, this French chocolate company can be found in more than sixty countries. It focuses on beans with avant-garde flavor profiles.
www.valrhona.com

Germany
Coppeneur: This German chocolate company is setting new standards in single-origin perfection, as a chocolate maker and a chocolate grower
www.coppeneurchocolate.com

Divine: Chocolate maker and pioneer in the Free Trade movement
www.diviniechocolateusa.com

Feodora: Considered one of Germany's top brands
Purchase at www.finedarkchocolate.com

Hachez: Exclusive, original recipes in a variety of eye-pleasing chocolate delights from chocolatier Joseph Emile Hachez, established in 1890
Purchase at www.mostlychocolate.com

Milka
www.milka.com

Reber
Purchase at www.mostlychocolates.com

Schokinag: Artisan chocolate company; the professional's choice for applications
www.schokinagna.com

Vivani: The world of sensual chocolate
www.vivani.de

Grenada
Grenada Chocolate: Organic chocolate and chocolate makers cooperative
www.grendachocolate.com

Holland
Droste: International Dutch chocolate company
www.droste.nl

Vivani: Premium organic chocolate
www.vivani.de

Israel
Max Brenner
www.maxbrenner.com

Italy
Amedei: Artisan fine chocolate made
  with rare cocoa beans
www.amadei-us.com

Cuba Venchi: Gourmet Italian
  chocolate
Purchase at www.chocolateworld
  wide.com

Domori: Single-origin chocolate
www.domori.com
Purchase at www.finedarkchocolate.
  com

Giraudi
Purchase at www.finedarkchocolate.
  com

Guido Gobino
Purchase at www.worldwide
  chocolate.com

L'Artigiano: Handcrafted Italian
  chocolates
www.lartigianoforli.it/eng

Slitti: Beautiful, delicious, Italian
  creations in the best stores around
  the world
www.slitti.it

Russia
Korkunov: Award-winning Russian
  chocolates
www.korkunov.ru

São Tomé
Claudio Corallo: Some of the
  most complex chocolates in the
  world
www.claudiocorallo.com

Spain
Chocovic
www.chocovic.es

Valor: Exquisite Spanish chocolate
  since 1881
Purchase at www.chocosphere.com

Switzerland
Camille Bloch: Traditional ambas-
  sadors of Swiss chocolate
www.camillebloch.ch

Felchlin: Exquisite chocolate for
  confectioners and chocolate
  masters
www.felchlin.com

Frey: Fine chocolates from
  Switzerland's large scale–production
  chocolate company
www.chocolate-frey.com

Lindt: Swiss chocolate for
  more than 125 years, available
  at retailers throughout
  the world
www.lindt.com

Terra Nostra: Gourmet organic
  chocolate
www.terranostrachocolate.com

Toblerone: Legendary triangular Swiss
  chocolate with honey and almond
  nougat
www.toblerone.com

United Kingdom
Cadbury: A leading global chocolate
  company
www.cadbury.com

Divine: Farmer-owned Fair Trade
  chocolate
www.divinechocolateusa.com

Green & Black's: Pioneers in ethical trading and organic chocolate
www.greenandblacks.com

L'artisan du Chocolat: Artisan of luxury chocolates
www.artisanduchocolat.com

Montezuma's: Innovative chocolate makers in the United Kingdom
www.montezumas.co.uk

United States

Amano: Artisanal chocolate hand-crafted to perfection
www.amanochocolate.com

Art Bar: Soy-free organic chocolate made with Swiss chocolate
www.ithacafinechocolates.com

Belvedere Chocolates: Traditional Belgian chocolates
www.belvederechocolates.com

The Chocolate Therapist: All-natural chocolate with nuts, berries, spices, and organic flavoring oils
www.thechocolatetherapist.com

Chocolove: Small-batch traditional European chocolate
www.chocolove.com

Chocopologie: Exquisite single-origin chocolate bars
www.knipschildt.net/chba.html

Chuao Chocolatier: Venezuelan artisan chocolatier produces a collection of all-natural chocolates inspired by ancient Maya recipes
www.chuaochocolatier.com

Dagoba: Exceptional 100% organic chocolate with many Fair Trade products
www.dagobachocolate.com

Ecco Bella: Maker of dark chocolate mask
www.eccobella.com

Endangered Species: 10 percent of profits is donated to species, habitat, and humanity
www.chocolatebar.com

Ghirardelli: America's longest continu-ally operating chocolate company
www.ghirardelli.com

Godiva: Exquisite filled chocolates
www.godiva.com

Guittard: Oldest family-owned and -operated chocolate company in the United States
www.guittard.com

La Tourangelle: Fine gourmet choco-lates produced with traditional methods
www.latourangelle.com

Lake Champlain Chocolates: Fresh, all-natural chocolates
www.lakechamplainchocolates.com

L'Artisan du Chocolat: Traditional French chocolates in Los Angeles
www.lartisanduchocolat.net

Marie Belle: Delicate, luxurious, chocolate confections
www.mariebelle.com

Nantucket Chocolates: Quality arti-sanal chocolates
www.nantucketchocolates.com

Newman's Own: Organic products for charity
www.newmansownorganics.com

Ojai Chocolat: Organic dairy-free, sugar-free chocolate made with agave nectar
www.chilihot-chocolat.com

Patric: Micro-batch fine dark chocolate
www.patric-chocolate.com

Rogue: Artisanal bean-to-bar chocolatier
www.roguechocolatier.com

Romolo: Chocolates made in the traditional Italian style
www.romolochocolates.com

Scharffenberger: Flavorful bean-to-bar chocolate maker
www.scharffenberger.com

Taza: Stone-ground organic chocolate
www.tazachocolate.com

Theo: Organic, Fair Trade, bean-to-bar chocolate
www.theochocolate.com

Vosges: Exotic chocolate made with ingredients from around the world
www.vosgeschocolate.com

Waialua Estate: Single-estate chocolate from Hawaii
Purchase at www.chocosphere.com

Venezuela
El Rey: Premium chocolate made in the traditional Venezuelan style
www.chocolates-elrey.com

Chocolate Research Web Sites
Launch into your own research program with these valuable sites.

All Chocolate
www.allchocolate.com

American Cocoa Research Institute
www.acri-cocoa.org

American Journal of Clinical Nutrition
www.ajcn.org

American Society for Nutrition
www.nutrition.org

CAOBISCO: Association of the Chocolate, Biscuit & Confectionery Industries of the EU
www.caobisco.com

Chocolate Manufacturers Association
www.candyusa.org

Cocoa Camino
www.cocoacamino.com (Fair Trade references)

Cocoa Merchants Association of America
www.cocoamerchants.com

Cocoa Research UK
www.cocoaresearch.com

Coffee, Sugar & Cocoa Exchange
www.csce.com

Dark Chocolate Research
www.darkchocolateresearch.com

Exploratorium: Type "chocolate" into any search engine to link with hundreds of articles and research reviews on chocolate
www.exploratorium.edu

Federation of Cocoa Conference
www.cocoafederation.com

Find Articles: Search for "chocolate" or "chocolate research"
www.findarticles.com

Food & Agriculture Organization of the United Nations
www.fao.org

International Cocoa Organization
www.icco.org

International Confectionery Association
www.international-confectionery.com

Journal of Agricultural and Food Chemistry
www.pubs.acs.org

Journal of American Medical Association
www.jama.ama-assn.org

Journal of Hypertension
www.jhypertension.com

Journal of Nutrition
www.jn.nutrition.org

Journal of the American Dietetic Association
www.eatright.org

Mars Information Site
www.chocolateinfo.com

National Confectioners Association
www.candyusa.com

National Institutes of Health
www.nih.gov

Web MD
www.webmd.com

World Cocoa Federation
www.worldcocoafoundation.org; Nutrition research: www .worldcocoafoundation.org/info center/document-research-center/ Cacao_HumanNutrition.asp

World Fair Trade Organization
www.wfto.com

Where to Purchase Couverture Chocolate

A "couverture" is a chocolate-making chocolate, sold in small chips or large blocks for melting. Obviously, starting with the right chocolate is the key to creating an amazing product. The following brands offer excellent couvertures.

To find the exact product, type "couvertures" into the search area of each Web site to locate the couvertures. To find more sources for couvertures, go to any search engine and type in "chocolate couvertures."

Amedei
www.chocolatetradingco.com

Cacao Barry
www.pastrychef.com

Callebaut
www.chocolatesource.com

Choco Vic
www.chocosphere.com

The Chocolate Therapist
www.TheChocolateTherapist.com

Dagoba
www.dagoba.com

Domori
www.chocosphere.com

El Rey
www.chocolatesource.com

Felchlin
www.felchlin.com

Fondue Chocolate
www.fondue4you.com/fountain_
    chocolate.cfm

Fountain Chocolate
www.chocolatefountainsatyourdoor
    .com

Galler
www.chocolatesource.com

Guittard
www.chocosphere.com

Michel Cluizel
www.chocolateworld.com

Plantations
www.cooksshophere.com

Santander
www.chocolate.com or www.choco
    sphere.com

Scharffenberger
www.scharffenberger.com or
    www.chocolateworld.com

Schokinag
www.worldpantry.com

Sugar Free
www.doninichocolate.com

Valhrona
www.chocolatesource.com or
    www.cooksshophere.com

Appendix B

Glycemic Index and Weight-Loss Summary

The glycemic index (GI) is a measure of the rate at which foods affect blood sugar levels. It's been around for quite a long time but gained popularity after the release of a book called *The Glucose Revolution: Life Plan* and, more recently, *The South Beach Diet*. Carbohydrates that break down quickly have a higher GI rating because they raise blood sugar levels quickly. Foods that take longer to break down have lower GI values because they raise blood sugar levels more slowly.

When blood sugar goes up, insulin is released into the bloodstream to bring sugar levels back down to a normal level. Insulin works double duty, however, because it's also the hormone that promotes the deposit of fat onto our bodies. Eating a diet filled with low GI foods keeps the insulin out of the bloodstream, and this helps keep the fat off. Fortunately, chocolate, especially when combined with nuts, comes in at a very low 33 on the glycemic index.

Glycemic index ratings range from 1 to 100. To keep blood sugar (and therefore insulin levels) at an ideal level, a person should try to eat foods that range between 0 and 60. If you eat a high and a low GI food together, however, the two will balance each other, and the net effect is a rating somewhere in between the two. I've listed a few popular snack choices in the following lists, but for a full glycemic index chart and a complete description of how you can use the index to help control weight, refer to *The Glucose Revolution: Life Plan*.

241

Following are GI ratings for sugars and sugar-free sweeteners.

Sweetener	GI Rating
Fructose	12
Glucose	82
Glucose tablets	146*
High fructose corn syrup	89*
Honey	77
Lactose	48
Maltitol	32
Maltodextrin	150*
Maltose	117
Maple syrup	73
Organic agave nectar	11
Sucrose	60
Xylitol	12

Source: International Tables of Glycemic Index and Glycemic Load Values; *Diabetes Care*, 2008

*Source: Blue Agave Nectar, www.BlueAgaveNectar.com

Note that maltitol is a popular sweetener used in sugar-free products, yet it still raises blood sugar more than fructose (fruit sugar) does. Also keep in mind that different GI sources report different values for the same food as a result of the way foods are tested and the amount consumed. This makes the entire process of figuring out the GI for any food confusing to say the least. But once you familiarize yourself with the various GI tables, you'll see that by eating whole, nonprocessed foods, nuts, and whole grains, you can easily avoid most of the high GI ratings.

Below are GI ratings for natural sweeteners.

Sweetener	GI Rating
Agave nectar, unrefined cane sugar	Low
Barley malt syrup, brown rice syrup	Medium
Dates, date sugar, fruit spreads, honey, maple syrup, apple syrup, birch syrup	High
Stevia leaf, oligofructose	Very low

Following are GI ratings for a variety of typical snacks.

Food	GI Rating
Bagel, 1 small plain (2 ounces)	72
Banana, 1 medium (5 ounces)	55
Blueberry muffin (2 ounces)	59
Cantaloupe, ¼ small	65
Cheerios, 1 cup (1 ounce)	74
Chocolate bar, 1½ ounces	49*
Chocolate milk, 8 ounces	34
Coca-Cola, 1 can	63
Cocoa Krispies, 1 cup	77
Cranberry juice, 8 ounces	52
Fettuccine, 1 cup	32
French fries, large (4.3 ounces)	75
Jelly beans, 10 large	80
Life cereal, 1 cup	66
Oat bran muffin	60
Oatmeal, old-fashioned, ½ cup	49
Peanut M&Ms, 1.7 ounces	33
Popcorn, 1¾ ounces	55
Pretzels, 1 ounce	83
Shortbread cookies, 4 pieces	64
Slim-Fast Chocolate Caramel meal replacement bar	77
Vermicelli, 1 cup	35
Watermelon, 1 cup	72
White bread, 1 slice	70
Yogurt, with sugar, 8 ounces	33

Source: International Tables of Glycemic Index and Glycemic Load Values; *Diabetes Care*, 2008

*The chocolate bar listed is not made from dark organic chocolate. I contacted the authors of *The Glucose Revolution* for information on dark chocolate, but it wasn't readily available. Yet they did note that all chocolate comes in quite low on the index because it contains fat, which slows its absorption into the bloodstream. A dark chocolate bar with nuts comes in even lower.

Following are the GI ratings for popular chocolate treats.

Chocolate	GI Rating
Cadbury milk chocolate	55
Chocolate Pop-Tarts	72
Dove dark chocolate	26
Kudos milk chocolate granola bar	56
Kudos whole-grain chocolate chip bar	70
Mars bar	70
Mars Cocovia chocolate almond bar	71
Milky Way bar	70
Milky Way Lite bar	50
Nutella hazelnut spread	29
Power Bar, chocolate	63
SmartZone chocolate bar, Hershey	15
SmartZone caramel bar, Hershey	20
Snickers bar	41
Twix bar	52
VO2 Max Energy bar, Mars	57

Source: International Tables of Glycemic Index and Glycemic Load Values, 2008

Some of the things we think of as ideal snacks, like Mars Cocovia or Kudos granola bars, actually raise blood sugar substantially. If you're heading out to hike or for a bike ride, these snacks work well because they help release insulin, and this helps the body release into the blood glycogen which can be used for energy. But if you're just sitting around the office and in need of a little treat, you're better off with a SmartZone bar, Nutella, or the Dove dark chocolate because they're low on the GI. Eating low-GI snacks also helps prevents the inevitable crash that follows a high-blood-sugar rush.

Appendix C

Chocolate Dictionary

alkalization   The use of potassium carbonate to make the chocolate darker, as well as to mellow its naturally acidic flavor. Alkalization also destroys some of the antioxidants in chocolate.

arriba   A type of bean from the Forestaro tree with a delicate and mild flavor. Considered one of the world's best cocoa beans.

cacahuatl   The Aztec word for *cacao bean*; the word *chocolate* is derived from this word.

cacao   Dried and fermented beans from which chocolate, cocoa powder, and cocoa butter are made.

cocoa butter   Fat that has been pressed out of the cocoa bean.

cocoa cake   Also called cocoa solids or press cake, cocoa cake is what is left once all of the cocoa butter has been pressed out of the cocoa beans. The cakes are generally pulverized into cocoa powder.

cocoa liquor   Shelled cocoa nibs that have been rolled back and forth between rollers until they become a liquid. It is a combination of the cocoa solids and the fats together, before they're separated.

cocoa nibs   Shelled, fermented beans that have broken into smaller pieces.

conching   Kneading the chocolate in huge vats with paddles, allowing it to be aerated. This process, named for the shell-shaped machine it's performed in, also emulsifies the fat, reduces the natural acidity of chocolate, develops the flavor, and smoothes the texture of chocolate.

couverture   Professional-quality chocolate, often delivered in small round bits and used for making chocolates. Various degrees of cocoa content are available.

Dutch process   Alkaline treatment of nibs prior to grinding. It darkens the chocolate and reduces the acidity of the natural cacao flavor (see alkalization).

emulsifier   Lecithin and polyglycerol polyricinoleate (PGPR) are the most common emulsifiers. Emulsifiers make chocolate more manageable by coating its solid particles, allowing them to move more easily.

enrobe   To coat the candy centers with chocolate.

fat bloom   A chalky white film on the surface of chocolate caused by the separation of cocoa butter from the rest of the chocolate.

ganache   Made with various proportions of chocolate and cream. Used for truffle centers and other chocolate desserts.

gianduja   Roasted hazelnuts and chocolate conched together.

lecithin   An emulsifier that is used to reduce the thickness of chocolate. This decreases the amount of cocoa butter that is needed to make a correctly textured chocolate.

mole poblano   A classic Mexican dish composed of turkey in a spicy, savory chocolate sauce.

press cake   Pressed cocoa powder after all of the cocoa butter has been extracted from the cocoa liquor. The cake can later be ground into cocoa powder.

seizing   The clumping and crystallization of melted chocolate when moisture touches it or when a cold liquid (or solid) is introduced.

sugar bloom   If chocolate is exposed to excessive moisture, the moisture evaporates and sugar crystals are left exposed, which can create an unattractive look.

vanillin   A form of artificial vanilla.

white chocolate   Made from cocoa butter, milk solids, sugar, soy lecithin, and vanilla. Top-quality white chocolate should have more than 20% cocoa butter.

winnowing   The process of removing the outer shells of the cacao beans during the manufacturing process, which is done by a large blower.

References

1. The Condensed History of Chocolate

Bennett, Alan. Out of the Amazon: Theobroma Cacao Enters the Genomic Era. *Trends in Plant Science* 8, no. 12 (December 2003): 561–563.

Chocolate Source. Chocolate: Rich in History. www.chocolatesource.com/history/index.asp.

Coe, Sophie D., and Michael D. Coe. *The True History of Chocolate*. New York: Thames and Hudson, 1996.

Jacobsen, Rowan. *Chocolate Unwrapped: The Surprising Health Benefits of America's Favorite Passion*. Montpelier, VT: Invisible Cities Press, 2003.

Wolfe, David, and Shazzie. *Naked Chocolate: The Astonishing Truth About the World's Greatest Food*. San Diego: Maul Brothers, 2005.

ZChocolat. World Cocoa Production. www.zchocolat.com/chocolate/chocolate/cocoa-production.asp.

2. From Cacao Tree to Chocolate Bar

Chocolate Source. Chocolate: The History of Chocolate. www.zchocolat.com/chocolate/chocolate/history-of-chocolate.asp.

Coe, Sophie D., and Michael D. Coe. *The True History of Chocolate*. New York: Thames and Hudson, 1996.

Gourmet Chocolate of the Month Club. www.chocolatemonthclub.com/pastfaqs.htm.

Jacobsen, Rowan. *Chocolate Unwrapped: The Surprising Health Benefits of America's Favorite Passion*. Montpelier, VT: Invisible Cities Press, 2003.

Scharffenberger, J., and R. Steinberg. *The Essence of Chocolate: Recipes for Baking and Cooking with Fine Chocolate*. New York: Hyperion, 2006.

Wolfe, David, and Shazzie. *Naked Chocolate: The Astonishing Truth About the World's Greatest Food*. San Diego: Maul Brothers, 2005.

ZChocolat. The Cocoa Tree. www.zchocolat.com/chocolate/chocolate/cocoa-tree.asp.

3. Healthy Investigation

Baba, S., M. Netsuke, A. Yasuda, et al. Plasma LDL and HDL Cholesterol and Oxidized LDL Concentrations Are Altered in Normal and Hypercholesterolemia Humans after Intake of Different Levels of Cocoa Powder. *American Society for Nutrition Journal of Nutrition* 137 (June 2007): 1436–1441.

Bauman College: Holistic Nutrition and Culinary Arts. www.BaumanCollege.com.

Candy USA. Cocoa and Chocolate Research Briefs: Analytical, Behavioral, Health and Nutrition Research, January–June 2009. http://nca.cms-plus.com/files/firsthalf2009cocoareasechbriefs.pdf.

Edwards, J., S. Villar, L. Fernando, C. de Oliveira, and M. Le Hyaric. Analytical Raman Spectroscopic Study of *Cacao* Seeds and Their Chemical Extracts. *Analytica Chimica Acta* 538 (2005): 175–180.

Enig, M. *Know Your Fats: The Complete Primer for Understanding the Nutrition of Fats, Oils and Cholesterol*. Silver Spring, MD: Bethesda Press, 2000.

Flavanols Key to Potential Chocolate Benefits. Science Daily. September 29, 2005. www.sciencedaily.com/releases/2005/09/050929081826.htm.

Free Radical Research Center. Medical College of Wisconsin. www.mcw.edu/FRRC/publications/2008Publications.htm.

Heo, J., and C. Lee. Epicatechin and Catechin in Cocoa Inhibit Amyloid B Protein- Induced Apoptosis. *Journal of Agriculture and Food Chemistry* 53, no. 5 (2005): 1445–1448.

Lee, K. W., Y. J. Kim, H. J. Lee, and C. Y. Lee. Cocoa Has More Phenolic Phytochemicals and a Higher Antioxidant Capacity Than Teas and Red Wine. *Journal of Agricultural and Food Chemistry* 51 (2003): 7292–7295.

Prescription Strength Chocolate, Revisited. Science News. www.sciencenews.org/view/generic/id/7075/title/Food_for_Thought.

Robbins, John. *Diet for a New America*. Tiburon, CA: H. J. Kramer, 1998.

Schneider, C., R. Cowles, C. Stuefer-Powell, and T. Carr. Dietary Stearic Acid Reduces Cholesterol Absorption and Increases Endogenous Cholesterol Excretion in Hamsters Fed Cereal-Based Diets. *Journal of Nutrition* 130 (2000): 1232–1238.

Sears, Barry. *The Zone*. New York: Regan Books, 1995.

Serafini, M., R. Bugianesi, G. Maiani, S. Valtuena, S. DeSantis, and A. Crozier. Plasma Antioxidants from Chocolate. *Nature* 424 (August 28, 2003): 1013.

Soon-Jae, J., and N. M. Betts. Copper Intakes and Consumption Patterns of Chocolate Foods as Sources of Copper for Individuals in the 1987–88 Nationwide Food Consumption Survey. *Nutrition Research* 16, no. 1 (January 1996): 41–52.

U.S. Department of Agriculture. www.ars.usda.gov/nutrientdata.

Wang, J. F., D. D. Schramm, R. R. Holt, et al. A Dose-Response Effect from Chocolate Consumption on Plasma Epicatechin and Oxidative Damage. *Journal of Nutrition* 1 (2000): 30.

Young, Robert O., and Shelly Redford. *The pH Miracle: Balance Your Diet, Reclaim Your Health.* New York: Warner Books, 2003.

4. Selecting the Proper Chocolate

Corn Syrup, High Fructose Corn Syrup. Free Dictionary. http://encyclopedia2 .thefreedictionary.com/Glucose+syrup.

Leventhal, Shari. High Fructose Corn Syrup: A Recipe for Hypertension. American Society of Nephrology, October 2009. Science Centric. www .sciencecentric.com/news/article.php?q=09103040-high-fructose-corn-syrup-recipe-hypertension.

Patent Storm. Film Coatings and Film Coating Compositions Based on Dextrin. February 19, 2002. www.PatentStorm.com.

Saudi Aramco World. Gum Arabic. March/April 2005. www .SaudiAramcoWorld.com.

Schroeter, H., R. Hold, T. Orozco, H. Schmitz, and C. Keen. Nutrition: Milk and Absorption of Dietary Flavanols. *Nature* 426 (December 18, 2003): 787–788.

Serafini, M., R. Bugianesi, G. Maiani, S. Valtuena, S. De Santis, and A. Crozier. Plasma Antioxidants from Chocolate. *Nature* 424 (August 28, 2003): 1013.

Winter, Ruth. *A Consumer's Dictionary of Food Additives.* New York: Three Rivers Press, 2004.

6. Chocolate Remedies

ADD/ADHD

Dean, Carolyn. *The Miracle of Magnesium: The Essential Nutrient That Works Wonders for Your Health and Energy.* New York: Ballantine Books, 2004.

Natural News. The Importance of Staving Off Magnesium Deficiency. May 21, 2008. www.naturalnews.com/magnesium_deficiency.html.

O'Shea, Timothy. "Minerals." The Doctor Within. www.thedoctorwithin .com/minerals/Minerals.

Allergies

About.com: Food Allergies. http://foodallergies.about.com/od/common foodallergies/f/chocolate.htm.

Usami, O., M. Belvisi, H. Patel, et al. Theobromine Inhibits Sensory Nerve Activation and Cough. *FASEF Journal* 19 (2005): 213–233.

Whole Health MD. Ginger. August 31, 2004. www.wholehealthmd.com.

Wolfe, David, and Shazzie. *Naked Chocolate: The Astonishing Truth About the World's Greatest Food.* San Diego: Maul Brothers, 2005.

Alzheimer's Disease

Alzheimer's Association. www.alz.org.

Bisson, J. F., A. Nejdi, P. Rozan, S. Hidalgo, R. Lalonde, and M. Messaoudi. Effects of Long-Term Administration of Cocoa Polyphenolic Extract (Acticoa powder) on Cognitive Performances in Aged Rats. *British Journal of Nutrition* 100, no. 1 (July 2008): 94–101.

Blueberries in the News. Wild About Blueberries. www.wildaboutberries.com/ healthy_stuff.htm.

Dai, Q., A. R. Borenstein, Y. Wu, J. C. Jackson, and E. B. Larson. Fruit and Vegetable Juices and Alzheimer's Disease: The Kame Project. *American Journal of Medicine* 119, no. 9 (September 2006): 751–759.

Heo, H. J., and C. Y. Lee. Epicatechin and Catechin in Cocoa Inhibit Amyloid Beta Protein Induced Apoptosis. *Journal of Agricultural and Food Chemistry* 53, no. 5 (March 9, 2005): 1445–1448.

University of Nottingham. Boosting Brain Power with Chocolate. February 2007. www.nottingham.ac.uk/public-affairs/press-releases/index.phtml? menu=pressreleases&code=BOOS-28/07&create_date=19-feb-2007.

Andropause

Geraci, Ron. Men's Health. December 25, 2000. www.timinvermont.com/ fitness/boosttes.htm.

Health Benefits of Macadamia Nuts. Maloha: The Hawaiian Company. www .maloha.com/healthbenefits.html.

Seidman, S. Normative Hypogonadism and Depression: Does "Andropause" Exist? *International Journal of Impotence Research* 18 (October 2006): 415–422.

Anemia

Dean, Carolyn. *The Miracle of Magnesium: The Essential Nutrient That Works Wonders for Your Health and Energy.* New York: Ballantine Books, 2004.

Kumari, M., S. Gupta, A. J. Lakshmi, and J. Prakash. Iron Bioavailability in Green Leafy Vegetables Cooked in Different Utensils. *Food Chemistry* 86, no. 2 (June 2004): 217–224.

Antiwrinkle Assistance

Gasser, P., E. Lati, L. Peno-Mazzarino, D. Bouzoud, L. Allgaert, and H. Bernaet. Cocoa Polyphenols and Their Influence on Parameters

Involved in Ex Vivo Skin Restructuring. *International Journal of Cosmetic Science* 30, no. 5 (October 2008): 339–345.

Stahl, W., U. Heinrich, K. Neukam, H. Tronnier, and H. Sies. Long-Term Ingestion of High Flavanol Cocoa Proves Photoprotection against UV-Induced Erythema and Improves Skin Condition in Women. American Society for Nutrition. *Journal of Nutrition* 136 (June 2006): 1565–1569.

Antioxidant Assistance

Geerligs, P. D., B. J. Brabin, and A. A. Omari. Food Prepared in Iron Cooking Pots as an Intervention for Reducing Iron Deficiency Anaemia in Developing Countries: A Systematic Review. *Journal of Human Nutrition and Dietetics* 16, no. 4 (August 2003): 275–281.

Hartman, Rustin. The Power of Antioxidants. *Breakthroughs in Health* 2, no. 1, (February 2007): 12–16.

Miller, Kenneth B., David A. Stuart, Nancy L. Smith, et al. Antioxidant Activity and Polyphenol and Procyanidin Contents of Selected Commercially Available Cocoa-Containing and Chocolate Products in the United States. *Journal of Agricultural and Food Chemistry* 54, no. 11 (May 2006): 4062–4068.

Nakamura, Jun, and James A. Swenberg. Endogenous Apurinic/Apyrimidinic Sites in Genomic DNA of Mammalian Tissues. *Cancer Research* 59 (June 1999): 2522–2526.

Science Daily. Hot Cocoa Tops Red Wine and Tea in Antioxidants: May Be a Healthier Choice. www.sciencedaily.com/releases/2003/11/031106051159.htm.

Vinson, J., J. Proch, P. Bose, et al. Chocolate Is a Powerful Ex Vivo and in Vivo Antioxidant, an Antiatherosclerotic Agent in an Animal Model, and a Significant Contributor to Antioxidants in the European and American Diets. *Journal of Agricultural Food and Chemistry* 54, no. 21 (October 2006): 8071–8076.

Whole Foods Supplements Guide. Sources of Antioxidants. www.whole-food-supplements-guide.com/sources-of-antioxidants.html.

Anxiety

Dean, Carolyn. *The Miracle of Magnesium: The Essential Nutrient That Works Wonders for Your Health and Energy.* New York: Ballantine Books, 2004.

Hoehn-Saric, Rudolph, Daniel R. McLeod, Frank Funderburk, and Pamela Kowalski. Somatic Symptoms and Physiologic Responses in Generalized Anxiety Disorder and Panic Disorder; *Archives of General Psychiatry* 61 (2004): 913–921.

Ross, Julia. *The Diet Cure.* New York: Penguin, 1999.

Arthritis

Abby, M. J., V. V. Patil, C. V. Vause, and P. L. Durhan. Repression of Calcitonin Gen-Related Peptide Expression in Trigeminal Neurons by a Theobroma Cacao Extract. *Journal of Enthnopharmacology* 115, no. 2 (January 17, 2008): 238–245.

Ahmed, Salahuddin, Naizhen Wang, Mathew Lalonde, Victor M. Goldberg, and Tariq M. Haqqi. Green Tea Polyphenol Epigallocatechin-3-gallate (EGCG) Differentially Inhibits Interleukin-1β-Induced Expression of Matrix Metalloproteinase-1 and -13 in Human Chondrocytes. *Journal of Pharmacology and Experimental Therapeutics* 308, no. 2, (November 2004): 767–773.

Arthritis.org. One in Three Americans Are Affected by Arthritis or Other Chronic Joint Problems. www.arthritis.org/media/newsroom/media-kits/Arthritis_Prevalence.pdf.

————.Water Exercise. www.arthritis.org/water-exercise.php.

Di Giuseppe, Romina, Augusto Di Castelnuovo, Floriana Centritto, et al. Regular Consumption of Dark Chocolate Is Associated with Low Serum Concentrations of C-Reactive Protein in a Healthy Italian Population. *Journal of Nutrition* 138 (October 2008): 1939–1945.

Miller, M., P. Bobrowski, S. Meenakshi, K. Gupta, and T. Haqqi. Chondroprotective Effects of a Proanthocyanidin Rich Amazonian Genonutrient Reflects Direct Inhibition of Matrix Metalloproteinase and Upregulation of IGF-1 Production by Human Chondrocytes. *Journal of Inflammation* 4 (August 2007): 16.

Porphyry's People. Nuts—the Surprising Health Benefits. September 7, 2004. www.vegan.org.nz.

Šarić, Ana, Sandra Sobočanec, Tihomir Balog, et al. Improved Antioxidant and Anti-inflammatory Potential in Mice Consuming Sour Cherry Juice. *Plant Foods for Human Nutrition* 64 (September 2009): 231–237.

Zold, D., P. Szodora, J. Gaal, et al. Vitamin D Deficiency in Undifferentiated Connective Tissue Disease. *Arthritis Research and Therapy* 10, no. 5 (October 2008): R123.

Asthma

Applied Health. Asthma. www.appliedhealth.com/nutri/page30.php.

Asthma World. Benefits of Proanthocyanidins—Antihistamine, Antioxidant and Anti-inflammatory. www.asthmaworld.org/flavonoid.htm.

Cosentino, Marco, Raffaella Bombelli, Ario Conti, et al. Antioxidant Properties and *in vitro* Immunomodulatory Effects of Peppermint (*Mentha x piperita l.*) Essential Oils in Human Leukocytes. *Journal of Pharmaceutical Sciences and Research* 1, no. 3 (2009): 33–43.

Rios, L., M. Gonthier, C. Remesv, et al. Chocolate Intake Increases Urinary Excretion of Polyphenol-Derived Phenolic Acids in Healthy Human Subjects. *American Journal of Clinical Nutrition* 77, no. 4 (April 2003): 912–918.

Tao of Herbs. Mint Comments and Uses. www.taoofherbs.com.

Blood Sugar Control

Almond Board of California. www.almondboard.com/HealthProfessionalsUK/
Pages/ConsumerSearchResults.aspx?k=diabetes.

Brand-Miller, Jennie, Johanna Burani, and Kaye Foster-Powell. *The Glucose
Revolution Life Plan: Discover How to Make the Glycemic Index the
Foundation for a Lifetime of Healthy Eating.* New York: Marlowe and
Company, 2000.

Cefalu, W., and F. Hu. Role of Chromium in Human Health and Diabetes.
American Diabetes Association, *Diabetes Care* 27, no. 11 (November
2004): 2741–2751.

Khan, A., M. Safdar, M. M. Ali Khan, K. N. Khattak, and R. Anderson.
Cinnamon Improves Glucose and Lipids of People with Type 2 Diabetes.
Diabetes Care 26 (December 2003): 3215–3218.

Tomaru, M., H. Takano, N. Osakabe, et al. Dietary Supplementation with
Cacao Liquor Proanthocyanidins Prevents Elevation of Blood Glucose Levels
in Diabetic Obese Mice. *Nutrition* 23, no. 4 (April 2007): 351–355.

Caffeine Withdrawal

De Camargo, M. C. R., and M. C. F. Toledo. HPLX Determination
of Caffeine in Tea, Chocolate Products and Carbonated Beverages.
Journal of the Science of Food and Agriculture 79, no.13 (1999):
1861–1864.

Wolfe, David, and Shazzie. *Naked Chocolate: The Astonishing Truth About the
World's Greatest Food.* San Diego: Maul Brothers, 2005.

Xocai: Healthy Chocolate. www.mxicorp.com/support/product.html.

Cancer

Bisson, J., M. Guardia-Llorens, S. Hidalgo, R. Pascale, and M. Messaoudi.
Protective Effect of Acticoa Powder, a Cocoa Polyphenolic Extract, on
Prostate Cancer in Wistar-Unilever Rats. *European Journal of Cancer
Prevention* 17, no. 1 (February 2008): 54–61.

D'Archivio, M., C. Santangelo, B. Scazzocchio, et al. Modulatory Effects of
Polyphenols on Apoptosis Induction: Relevance for Cancer Prevention.
International Journal of Molecular Science 9, no. 3 (March 2008):
213–228.

Mahmoud, N., A. Carothers, D. Grunberger, et al. Plant Phenolics Decrease
Intestinal Tumors in an Animal Model of Familial Adenomatous Polyposis.
Carcinogenesis 21, no. 5 (May 2000): 921–927.

Shklar, G., et al. The Effectiveness of a Mixture of Beta-Carotene, Alpha-
Tocopherol, Glutathione, and Ascorbic Acid for Cancer Prevention.
Nutrition and Cancer 20 (1993): 145–151.

Cataracts

Blue Mountain Eye Study. Center for Vision Research, 1992–2002. www.cvr
.org.au/bmes.htm.

Mayo Clinic. Cataracts. May 2008. www.mayoclinic.com/ health/cataracts/ DS00050/DSECTION=causes.

Tan, A. G., P. Mitchell, V. M. Flood, et al. Antioxidant Nutrient Intake and the Long-Term Incidence of Age-Related Cataracts: The Blue Mountains Eye Study. *American Journal of Clinical Nutrition* 87, no. 6 (June 2008): 1899–1905.

Cavities

Oshima, T., and H. Osaka. Utility of Chocolate/Cocoa. Dental Caries Inhibitory Effect of Cacao Extract. *Shoku no Kagaku* 252 (1999): 46–49.

Ott, Jonathan. *The Cacahuatl Eater: Ruminations of an Unabashed Chocolate Addict.* Vashon, WA: Natural Products, 1985.

Srikanth, R. K., N. D. Shashikiran, and V. V. Subba Reddy. Chocolate Mouth Rinse: Effect on Plaque Accumulation and Mutants Streptococci Counts When Used by Children. *Journal of Indian Society of Pedodontics & Preventive Dentistry* 26, no. 2 (April–June 2008): 67–70.

Chronic Fatigue

Khan, A., M. Safdar, M. M. Ali, Khan, K. N. Khattak and R. Anderson. Cinnamon Improves Glucose and Lipids of People with Type 2 Diabetes. *Diabetes Care* 26 (December 2003): 3215–3218.

Sathyapalan, T., P. Campion, S. Beckett, A. Ribgy, and S. Atkin. High Cocoa Polyphenol Rich Chocolate Improves the Symptoms of Chronic Fatigue. *Endocrine Abstracts* 12 (November 2006): 68.

Stampfer, M. J., F. Hu, J. Manson, E. Rimm, and W. Willete. Primary Prevention of Coronary Heart Disease in Women through Diet and Lifestyle. *New England Journal of Medicine* 343 (July 2000): 16–22.

Constipation

Body Mind Revival. Body Detox: The Process to Purify Your Life, Mind and Soul. www.bodymindrevival.com/category/body-detox.

California Almond Board. Trust Your Gut. www.almondboard.com/ Consumer/HealthandNutrition/Pages/Prebiotics.aspx.

Dillinger, T., P. Barriga, S. Escarcega, M. Jimenez, D. S. Lowe, and L. Grivetti. Food of the Gods: Cure for Humanity? A Cultural History of the Medicinal and Ritual Use of Chocolate. *Journal of Nutrition* 130 (2000): 2057S–S072S.

Cough

Schroeter, H., R. Hold, T. Orozco, H. Schmitz, and C. Keen. Nutrition: Milk and Absorption of Dietary Flavanols. *Nature* 426 (December 2003): 787–788.

Tealand.com. www.tealand.com/Cold_Flu_Traditional_Medicinals.aspx.

Usami O., M. Belvisi, H. Patel, et al. Theobromine Inhibits Sensory Nerve Activation and Cough. *FASEB Journal* 19 (2005): 213–233.

Cramps
Wolfe, David, and Shazzie. *Naked Chocolate: The Astonishing Truth About the World's Greatest Food.* San Diego: Maul Brothers, 2005.

Depression
Beltrama, M., and D. Piomelli. Trick or Treat from Food Endocannabinoids. *Nature* 396 (December 1998): 636–637.

Dried Fruit Information Services. About Dried Fruit: Nutritional Information. www.driedfruit-info.com.

Edwards, J., S. Villar, L. Fernando, C. de Oliveira, and M. Le Hyaric. Analytical Raman Spectroscopic Study of Cacao Seeds and Their Chemical Extracts. *Analytica Chimica Acta* 538 (2005):175–180.

Marino, Jon. Prescription Strength Chocolate. *Science News* (February 2004).

Romolo Chocolates. Here's to Your Health and Happiness: Toasting the Benefits and Pleasures of Chocolate. www.romolochocolates.com.

Ross, Julia. *The Diet Cure.* New York: Penguin, 1999.

Wolfe, David, and Shazzie. *Naked Chocolate: The Astonishing Truth About the World's Greatest Food.* San Diego: Maul Brothers, 2005.

Diabetes
Atkinson, F. S., K. Foster-Powell, and J. C. Brand-Miller. International Tables of Glycemic Index and Glycemic Load Values: 2008. *Diabetes Care* 31, no. 12 (2008).

Balzer, Jan, Tienush Rassaf, Christian Heiss, et al. Sustained Benefits in Vascular Function Through Flavanol-Containing Cocoa in Medicated Diabetic Patients. *Journal of the American College of Cardiology* 51 (January 2008): 2141–2149.

Brand-Miller, Jennie, Johanna Burani, and Kaye Foster-Powell. *The Glucose Revolution Life Plan: Discover How to Make the Glycemic Index the Foundation for a Lifetime of Healthy Eating.* New York: Marlowe and Company, 2000.

Cruise, Jorge. *8 Minutes in the Morning: A Simple Way to Shed Up to 2 Pounds a Week—Guaranteed.* New York: St. Martin's Press, 2001.

Outsmart Diabetes special issue. *Prevention Guide.* New York: Rodale/St. Marten's Press, 2008.

Rosen, Kelli. The Sugar Debate. *Delicious Living*, February 1, 2008.

Doggy Danger
Bistner, S., R. Ford, and M. Raffe. *Kirk and Bistner's Handbook of Veterinary Procedures and Emergency Treatment.* Philadelphia: W. B. Saunders, February 2000.

Dalzell, Bonnie. Notes on Chocolate Toxicity in Dogs. *NetPet Magazine.* http://netpet.batw.net/articles/choc.tox.html.

Gans, J., R. Korson, M. Cater, and C. Ackerly. Effects of Short-Term and Long-Term Theobromine Administration to Male Dogs. *Science Direct.* August 1979. www.ScienceDirect.com.

Emphysema

E Health MD. Living with Emphysema. www.ehealthmd.com/library/Emphysema/EMP_living.html.

Heiss, C., P. Kleinbongard, A. Dejam, et al. Acute Consumption of Flavanol-Rich Cocoa and the Reversal of Endothelial Dysfunction in Smokers. *Journal of American College of Cardiology* 46, no. 7 (October 2005): 1276–1283.

Energy Loss

Cagindi, Ozlem, and Sehmi Ottles. The Health Benefits of Chocolate Enrichment with Dried Fruits. *Acta Scientarium Polonorum, Technologia Alimentaria* 8, no. 4 (2009): 63–69.

Coe, Sophie D., and Michael D. Coe. *The True History of Chocolate.* New York: Thames and Hudson, 1996.

Colgan, Michael. *Sports Nutrition Guide: Minerals, Vitamins, and Antioxidants for Athletes.* Vancouver, Canada: Apple Publishing Company, 2002.

Dean, Carolyn. *The Miracle of Magnesium: The Essential Nutrient That Works Wonders for Your Health and Energy.* New York: Ballantine Books, 2004.

Fiber Shortage

Kamiwaki, T, K. Tsuji, and Y. Nakagawa. Effects of Dietary Fiber from Cacao Bean on Blood Pressure and Lipid Metabolism in Spontaneously Hypertensive Rats. *Journal of the Japanese Society for Food Science and Technology* 26, no. 9 (1999): 581–586.

Wolfe, David, and Shazzie. *Naked Chocolate: The Astonishing Truth About the World's Greatest Food.* San Diego: Maul Brothers, 2005.

Fibromyalgia

Holistic Online.com. Fibromyalgia: Nutrition and Diet. www.holisticonline.com/remedies/cfs/fib_nutrition.htm.

Lipski, E. *Digestive Wellness: How to Strengthen the Immune System and Prevent Disease Through Healthy Digestion.* New York: McGraw Hill, 2005.

Murray, Michael T. *Encyclopedia of Nutritional Supplements: The Essential Guide for Improving Your Health Naturally.* Rocklin, CA: Prima, 1996.

Flatulence

Coe, Sophie D., and Michael D. Coe. *The True History of Chocolate.* New York: Thames and Hudson, 1996.

Murdock, Linda. *A Busy Cook's Guide to Spices: How to Introduce New Flavors to Everyday Meals.* Denver, CO: Bellwether Books, 2007.

Spirling, Lucy, and Ian Daniels. Botanical Perspectives on Health: Peppermint, More Than Just an After Dinner Mint. *Journal of the Royal Society for the Promotion of Health* 121, no. 1 (2001): 62–63.

Vitacost.com. www.vitacost.com/Alvita-Caffeine-Free-Tea-Peppermint-Leaf.

Food Cravings

Erskine, J. A. Resistance Can Be Futile: Investigating Behavioural Rebound. *Appetite* 50, no. 2–3 (March–May 2008): 415–421.

Seligson, F. H., D. A. Krummel, and J. L. Apgar. Patterns of Chocolate Consumption. *American Journal of Clinical Nutrition* 60 (December 1994): 1060S–1064S.

Waterhouse, Debra. *Why Women Need Chocolate: Eat What You Crave to Look Good and Feel Great.* Portland, ME: Waterhouse, 1995.

Yuan, C., L. Dey, J. Xie, and H. Aung. Gastric Effects of Galanin and Its Interaction with Leptin on Brainstem Neuronal Activity. *Journal of Pharmacology and Experimental Therapeutics* 301, no. 2 (May 2002): 488–493.

Going to the Dark Side

Vinson, Joe, J. Proch, J. Zublik, and L. Zubik. Phenol Antioxidant Quantity and Quality in Foods: Cocoa, Dark Chocolate, and Milk Chocolate. *Journal of Agricultural and Food Chemistry* 47, no. 12 (1999): 4821–4824.

Headache

Dean, Carolyn. *The Miracle of Magnesium: The Essential Nutrient That Works Wonders for Your Health and Energy.* New York: Ballantine Books, 2004.

Gourley, L. A Double-Blind Provocative Study of Chocolate as a Trigger of Headache. *Cephalalgia* 17, no. 8 (December 1997): 855–862.

Pearson, D., T. Paglieroni, D. Rein, et al. The Effects of Flavanols-Rich Cocoa and Aspirin on Ex Vivo Platelet Function. *Thrombosis Research* 106, no. 4–5 (May 2002): 191–197.

Rein, D., T. G. Paglieroni, T. Wun, et al. Cocoa Inhibits Platelet Activation and Function. *American Journal of Nutrition* 72 (2000): 30–35.

Wang-Polagruto, Janice F., Amparo C. Villablanca, John A. Polagruto, et al. Chronic Consumption of Flavanol-Rich Cocoa Improves Endothelial Function and Decreases Vascular Cell Adhesion Molecule in Hypercholesterolemic Postmenopausal Women. *Journal of Cardiovascular Pharmacology* 47, Supplement 2 (June 2006): S177–S186.

Heartbreak

Sabelli, H., P. Fink, J. Fawcett, and C. Tom. Sustained Antidepressant Effect of PEA Replacement. *Journal of Neuropsychiatry Clinical Neuroscience* 8, no. 2 (1996): 168–71.

Szabo, A., E. Billett, and J. Turner. Phenylethylamine: A Possible Link to the Antidepressant Effects of Exercise? *British Journal of Sports Medicine* 35, no. 5 (October 2001): 342–343.

Heart Disease

Almond Board of California. Almonds—at the Heart of a Healthful Diet. www.almondboard.com/HealthProfessionalsUK/nutritionandresearch/Pages/HeartHealth.aspx.

Bearden, M., D. Rein, D. Pearson, et al. Potential Cardiovascular Health Benefits of Procyanidins Present in Chocolate and Cocoa. American Chemical Society Symposium Series 754, no. 19 (2000): 177–186.

De Nigris, F., S. Williams-Ignarrot, L. Lermant, et al. Beneficial Effects of Pomegranate Juice on Oxidation-Sensitive Genes and Endothelial Nitric Oxide Synthase Activity at Sites of Perturbed Shear Stress. *Proceedings of the National Academy of Sciences* 102, no. 13 (March 29, 2005): 4896–4901.

Dietrich, Rein, Debra Pearson, Teresa Paglieroni, Theodore Wun, Harold Schmitz, and Carl Keen. Cocoa Inhibits Platelet Activation and Function. *American Journal of Clinical Nutrition* 72 (July 2000): 30–35.

Hannum, Sandra M., Harold H. Schmitz, and Carl L. Keen. Chocolate: A Heart-Healthy Food: Show Me the Science! *Nutrition Today* 37, no. 3 (May/June 2002): 103–109.

Rein, D., S. Lotito, R. Holt, C. Keen, H. Schmitz, and C. Fraga. Epicatechin in Human Plasma: In Vivo Determination and Effect of Chocolate Consumption on Plasma Antioxidant Capacity. *Journal of Nutrition* 130 (2000): 2109S–2114S.

Schmitz, H., and L. Romanczyk. Proanthocyanidins: Biological Activities Associated with Human Health. *Pharmaceutical Biology* 42, no. S1 (2004): 2–20.

Shiina, Y., N. Funabashi, K. Lee, et al. Acute Effect of Oral Flavonoid-Rich Dark Chocolate Intake on Coronary Circulation, as Compared with Non-Flavonoid White Chocolate, by Transthoracic Doppler Echocardiography in Healthy Adults. *International Journal of Cardiology* 131, no. 3 (January 24, 2009): 424–429.

Steinberg, Francene, Monica M. Bearden, and Carl L. Keen. Cocoa and Chocolate Flavonoids: Implications for Cardiovascular Health. *Journal of the American Dietetic Association* 103, no. 2 (February 2003): 215–23.

Talan, Jamie. Dark Chocolate May Protect Your Heart. *Atlanta Journal Constitution*, June 2, 2004.

Wang-Polagruto, Janice F., Amparo C. Villablanca, et al. Chronic Consumption of Flavanol-Rich Cocoa Improves Endothelial Function and Decreases Vascular Cell Adhesion Molecule in Hypercholesterolemic Postmenopausal Women. *Journal of Cardiovascular Pharmacology* 47, no. 2 (June 2006): S177–S186.

High Blood Pressure / Hypertension

Allen, R. R., L. Carson, C. Kwik-Uribe, E. M. Evans, and J. W. Erdman Jr. Daily Consumption of a Dark Chocolate Containing Flavanols and Added Sterol Esters Affects Cardiovascular Risk Factors in a Normointensive Population with Elevated Cholesterol. *Journal of Nutrition* 138 (April 2008): 725–731.

Al-Mahroos, F., K. Roomi, and P. McKein. Relation of High Blood Pressure to Glucose Intolerance, Plasma Lipids and Educational Status in an Arabian Gulf Population. *International Journal of Epidemiology* 29 (2000): 71–76.

Bayard, V., F. Chamorro, J. Motta, and N. Hollenberg. Does Flavanol Intake Influence Mortality from Nitric Oxide-Dependent Processes? Ischemic Heart Disease, Stroke, Diabetes Mellitus, and Cancer in Panama. *International Journal of Medical Sciences* 4 (2007): 53–58.

Dietrich, Rein, Debra Pearson, Teresa Paglieroni, Theodore Wun, Harold Schmitz, and Carl Keen. Cocoa Inhibits Platelet Activation and Function. *American Journal of Clinical Nutrition* 72, no. 1 (July 2000): 30–35.

Sies, N., C. Kwik-Uribe, C. Schmitz, and M. Kel. Epicatechin Mediates Beneficial Effects of Flavanol Rich Cocoa on Vascular Function in Humans. *Proceedings of the National Academy of Sciences of the USA* 130 (2006): 1024–1029.

High Cholesterol

Allen, R. R., L. Carson, C. Kwik-Uribe, E. M. Evans, and J. W. Erdman Jr. Daily Consumption of a Dark Chocolate Containing Flavanols and Added Sterol Esters Affects Cardiovascular Risk Factors in a Normotensive Population with Elevated Cholesterol. *Journal of Nutrition* 138 (April 2008): 725–731.

Aviram, M., M. Rosenblat, D. Gaitini, et al. Pomegranate Juice Consumption for 3 Years by Patients with Carotid Artery Stenosis Reduces Common Carotid Intima-Media Thickness, Blood Pressure and LDL Oxidation. *Clinical Nutrition* 23, no. 3 (July 2004): 423–433.

Bonanome, A., and S. M. Grundy. Effect of Dietary Stearic Acid on Plasma Cholesterol and Lipoprotein Levels. *New England Journal of Medicine* 318, no. 19 (May 1988): 1244–1248.

Di Giuseppe, Romina Augusto Di Castelnuovo, Floriana Centritto, et al. Regular Consumption of Dark Chocolate Is Associated with Low Serum Concentrations of C-Reactive Protein in a Healthy Italian Population. *Journal of Nutrition* 138 (October 2008): 1939–1945.

Dietrich, Rein, Debra Pearson, Teresa Paglieroni, Theodore Wun, Harold Schmitz, and Carl Keen. Cocoa Inhibits Platelet Activation and Function. *American Journal of Clinical Nutrition* 72 (July 2000): 30–35.

Edwards J., S. Villar, L. Fernando, C. de Oliveira, and M. Le Hyaric. Analytical Raman Spectroscopic Study of *Cacao* Seeds and Their Chemical Extracts. *Analytica Chimica Acta* 538 (2005): 175–180.

Enig, M. *Know Your Fats: The Complete Primer for Understanding the Nutrition of Fats, Oils and Cholesterol.* Silver Spring, MD: Bethesda Press, 2008.

Foreman, Judy. Cinnamon Joins Cholesterol Battle. *Boston Globe.* August 24, 2004.

Jacobsen, Rowan. *Chocolate Unwrapped: The Surprising Health Benefits of America's Favorite Passion.* Montpelier, VT: Invisible Cities Press, 2003.

Schneider, Craig L., Russell L. Cowles, Cindy L. Stuefer-Powell, and Timothy P. Carr. Dietary Stearic Acid Reduces Cholesterol Absorption and Increases Endogenous Cholesterol Excretion in Hamsters Fed Cereal-Based Diets. *Journal of Nutrition* 130 (2000): 1232–1238.

Wan, Y., J. Vinson, T. Etherton, J. Proch, S. Lazarus, and P. Kris-Etherton. Effects of Cocoa Powder and Dark Chocolate on LDL Oxidative Susceptibility and Prostaglandin Concentrations in Humans. *American Journal of Clinical Nutrition* 74, no. 5 (November 2001): 596–602.

Wu, W., Y. Kang, N. Wang, J. Hei-Jan, and T. Want. Sesame Ingestion Affects Sex Hormones, Antioxidant Status, and Blood Lipids in Postmenopausal Women. *Journal of Nutrition* 136, no. 5 (May 2006): 1270–1275.

Hyperglycemia/Hypoglycemia

Atkinson, F. S., K. Foster-Powell, and J. C. Brand-Miller. International Tables of Glycemic Index and Glycemic Load Values: 2008. *Diabetes Care* 31, no. 12 (2008).

Brand-Miller, Jennie, Johanna Burani, and Kaye Foster-Powell. *The Glucose Revolution Life Plan: Discover How to Make the Glycemic Index the Foundation for a Lifetime of Healthy Eating.* New York: Marlowe and Company, 2001.

Immune Deficiency

Kurahashi, N., M. Inoie, M. Iwasaki, Y. Tanaka, M. Mizokami, and S. Tsugane. Vegetable, Fruit and Antioxidant Nutrient Consumption and Subsequent Risk of Hepatocellular Carcinoma: A Prospective Cohort Study in Japan. *British Journal of Cancer* 100 (2009): 181–184.

Porter, Leah H. Benefits of Cocoa Polyphenols. *The Manufacturing Confectioner* (June 2006).

Impotence

Akunyili, Dora. Viagra Works, but Chocolate Works Better. *Sexual Reproductive* 5, no. 16 (October 2006): 21.

Edwards, J., S. Villar, L. Fernando, C. de Oliveira, and M. Le Hyaric. Analytical Raman Spectroscopic Study of *Cacao* Seeds and Their Chemical Extracts. *Analytica Chimica Acta* 538 (2005): 175–180.

Wolfe, David, and Shazzie. *Naked Chocolate: The Astonishing Truth About the World's Greatest Food.* San Diego: Maul Brothers, 2005.

Wu, W., Y. Kang, N. Wang, J. Hei-Jan, and T. Want. Sesame Ingestion Affects Sex Hormones, Antioxidant Status, and Blood Lipids in Postmenopausal Women. *Journal of Nutrition* 136, no. 5 (May 2006): 1270–1275.

Infertility

Fraga, C. G., P. A. Motchnik, M. K. Shigenaga, H. J. Helbock, R. A. Jacob, and B. N. Ames. Ascorbic Acid Protects against Endogenous Oxidative DNA Damage in Human Sperm. *Proceedings of the National Academy of Sciences* 88 (December 1991): 11003–11006.

Mendiola, J., A. Torres-Canter, J. Moreno-Grau, et al. Food Intake and Its Relationship with Semen Quality: A Case-Control Study. *Journal of the American Society for Reproductive Medicine* 91, no. 3 (March 2009): 812–818.

Murray, Michael T. *Encyclopedia of Nutritional Supplements: The Essential Guide for Improving Your Health Naturally.* Rocklin, CA: Prima Publishing, 1996.

Insomnia

Kiyoshi, M., O. Shiro, N. Hiromi, and Y. Etsuko. Correlation between the Indices of Autonomic Nervous System and Mood after Drinking Chamomile Tea. *Japanese Journal of Biofeedback Research* 28 (2001): 61–70.

Plants and Potions. Can't Sleep? www.plantsandpotions.com/category/herbs-and-spices.

Ringdahl, E., S. Pereira, and J. Delzell. Treatment of Primary Insomnia. *Journal of the American Board of Family Practice* 17 (2004): 212–219.

Lack of Sexual Desire

Edwards, J., S. Villar, L. Fernando, C. de Oliveira, and M. Le Hyaric. Analytical Raman Spectroscopic Study of *Cacao* Seeds and Their Chemical Extracts. *Analytica Chimica Acta* 538 (2005): 175–180.

Salonia, A., F. Fabbri, G. Zanni, et al. Chocolate and Women's Sexual Health: An Intriguing Correlation. *Journal of Sexual Medicine* 3, no. 3 (February 2006): 476–482.

Wolfe, David, and Shazzie. *Naked Chocolate: The Astonishing Truth About the World's Greatest Food.* San Diego: Maul Brothers, 2005.

Lactose Intolerance

Lee, C., and C. Hardy. Cocoa Feeding and Human Lactose Intolerance. *American Journal of Clinical Nutrition* 49 (1989): 840–844.

Life Expectancy

Fraser, G. E., and D. J. Shavlik. Ten Years of Life: Is It a Matter of Choice? *Archives of Internal Medicine* 161, no. 13 (July 9, 2001): 1645–1652.

Key, T. J., G. E. Fraser, M. Thorogood, et al. Mortality in Vegetarians and Nonvegetarians: Detailed Findings from a Collaborative Analysis of 5 Prospective Studies. *American Journal of Clinical Nutrition* 70, no. 3 Suppl. (September 1999): 516S–524S.

Lee, I., and R. Paffenbarger. Life Is Sweet: Candy Consumption and Longevity. *British Medical Journal* 317 (1998): 1683–1684.

Macular Degeneration

Dean, Carolyn. *The Miracle of Magnesium: The Essential Nutrient That Works Wonders for Your Health and Energy.* New York: Ballantine Books, 2004.

Murray, Michael T. *The Encyclopedia of Healing Foods: The Essential Guide for Improving Your Health Naturally.* New York: Atria Books, 2005.

Seddon, J., J. Cote, and B. Rosner. Progression of Age-Related Macular Degeneration. Association with Dietary Fat, Transunsaturated Fat, Nuts and Fish Intake. *Archives of Ophthalmology* 121 (2003): 1728–1737.

Memory Loss

Bisson, J. F., A. Nejdi, P. Rozan, S. Hidalgo, R. Lalonde, and M. Messaoudi. Effects of Long-Term Administration of Cocoa Polyphenolic Extract (Acticoa powder) on Cognitive Performances in Aged Rats. *British Journal of Nutrition* 100, no. 1 (July 2008): 94–101.

Crews, W., D. Harrison, and J. Wright. A Double-Blind, Placebo-Controlled, Randomized Trial of the Effects of Dark Chocolate and Cocoa on Variables Associated with Neuropsychological Functioning and Cardiovascular Health: Clinical Findings from a Sample of Healthy, Cognitively Intact Older Adults. *American Journal of Clinical Nutrition* 87, no. 4 (April 2008): 872–880.

University of Nottingham. Boosting Brain Power with Chocolate. February 2007. www.nottingham.ac.uk/public-affairs/press-releases/index.phtml?menu=pressreleases&code=BOOS-28/07&create_date=19-feb-2007.

Menopause

Dean, Carolyn. *The Miracle of Magnesium: The Essential Nutrient That Works Wonders for Your Health and Energy.* New York: Ballantine Books, 2004.

Ford, E., and A. Mokdad. Dietary Magnesium Intake in a National Sample of US Adults. *Journal of Nutrition* 133 (September 2003): 2879–2882.

Hormone Foundation. Menopause: Managing Your Body's Changes. March 2006. www.hormone.org/Resources/upload/menopause_managing_your_body.pdf.

Mayo Clinic. Hot Flashes: Minimize Discomfort during Menopause. June 12, 2007. www.mayoclinic.com/health/hot-flashes/HQ01409.

Wang-Polagruto, Janice F., Amparo C. Villablanca, John A. Polagruto, et al. Chronic Consumption of Flavanol-Rich Cocoa Improves Endothelial Function and Decreases Vascular Cell Adhesion Molecule in Hypercholesterolemic Postmenopausal Women. *Journal of Cardiovascular Pharmacology* 47, Suppl 2 (June 2006): S177–S186.

Ziaei, S., A. Kazemnejad, and M. Zareai. Effect of Vitamin E on Hot Flashes in Post Menopausal Women. *Gynecologic Obstetric Investigation* 64 (2007): 204–207.

Mental Performance

Bisson, J. F., A. Nejdi, P. Rozan, S. Hidalgo, R. Lalonde, and M. Messaoudi. Effects of Long-Term Administration of Cocoa Polyphenolic Extract (Acticoa powder) on Cognitive Performances in Aged Rats. *British Journal of Nutrition* 100, no. 1 (July 2008): 94–101.

Nurk, E., H. Refsum, C. A. Drevon, et al. Intake of Flavonoid-Rich Wine, Tea, and Chocolate by Elderly Men and Women Is Associated with Better

Cognitive Test Performance. *Journal of Nutrition* 139, no. 1 (January 2009): 120–127.

University of Nottingham. Boosting Brain Power with Chocolate. February 2007. www.nottingham.ac.uk/public-affairs/press-releases/index.phtml? menu=pressreleases&code=BOOS-28/07&create_date=19-feb-2007.

Wheeling Jesuit University. Professor Finds That Chocolate Consumption Enhances Cognitive Performance. April 29, 2006. www.wju.edu/about/ adm_news_story.asp?iNewsID=2043.

Mood Swings

Edwards, J., S. Villar, L. Fernando, C. de Oliveira, and M. Le Hyaric. Analytical Raman Spectroscopic Study of *Cacao* Seeds and Their Chemical Extracts. *Analytica Chimica Acta* 538 (2005):175–180.

Wolfe, David, and Shazzie. *Naked Chocolate: The Astonishing Truth About the World's Greatest Food.* San Diego: Maul Brothers, 2005.

Nausea/Speaking in Public

Home Remedy Reference Center. www.home-remedy.org/home-remedy-for-nausea.html.

Murray, Michael T. *The Encyclopedia of Healing Foods: The Essential Guide for Improving Your Health Naturally.* New York: Atria Books, 2005.

Osteoporosis

Murray, Michael T. *The Encyclopedia of Healing Foods: The Essential Guide for Improving Your Health Naturally.* New York: Atria Books, 2005.

————. *Encyclopedia of Nutritional Supplements: The Essential Guide for Improving Your Health Naturally.* Rocklin, CA: Prima Publishing, 1996.

O'Shea, Timothy. "Minerals." The Doctor Within. www.thedoctorwithin .com/minerals/Minerals.

Schroeter, H., R. Hold, T. Orozco, H. Schmitz, and C. Keen. Nutrition: Milk and Absorption of Dietary Flavanols. *Nature* 426 (December 18, 2003): 787–788.

PMS

Dean, Carolyn. *The Miracle of Magnesium: The Essential Nutrient That Works Wonders for Your Health and Energy.* New York: Ballantine Books, 2004.

Natural News. The Importance of Staving Off Magnesium Deficiency. May 21, 2008. www.naturalnews.com/magnesium_deficiency.html.

Ross, Julia. *The Diet Cure.* New York: Penguin, 1999.

Somer, Elizabeth. Crazy for Chocolate. Elizabeth Somer.com. August 13, 2004.

Pregnancy

Raikkonen, K., A. Personen, A. Jarvenpaa, and T. Strandberg. Sweet Babies: Chocolate Consumption during Pregnancy and Infant Temperament at Six Months. *Early Human Development* 76, no. 2 (February 2004): 139–145.

Triche, Elizabeth W., Laura M. Grosso, Kathleen Belanger, et al. Chocolate Consumption in Pregnancy and Reduced Likelihood of Preeclampsia. *Epidemiology* 19, no. 3 (May 2008): 459–464.

Prostate Cancer

Bisson, Jean-François, Maria-Alba Guardia-Llorens, Sophie Hidalgo, Pascale Rozan, and Michaël Messaoudi. Protective Effect of Acticoa Powder, a Cocoa Polyphenolic Extract, on Prostate Carcinogenesis in Wistar-Unilever Rats. *European Journal of Cancer Prevention* 17, no. 1 (February 2008): 54–61.

Hu, G, J. Tuomilehto, E. Pukkala, et al. Joint Effects of Coffee Consumption and Serum Gamma-Glutamyltransferase on the Risk of Liver Cancer. *Hepatology* 48, no. 1 (July 2008): 129–136.

Larsson, S., and A. Wolk. Coffee Consumption and Risk of Liver Cancer: A Meta-Analysis. *Gastroenterology* 132, no. 5 (May 2007): 1740–1745.

Nkondjock, A. Coffee Consumption and the Risk of Cancer. An Overview. *Cancer Letters* 277, no. 2 (May 2009): 121–125.

Wilson, K., J. Kasperzyk, J. Stark, et al. Coffee Consumption Associated with Reduced Risk of Advanced Prostate Cancer. *Cancer Prevention Research* 3, Suppl 1 (January 2010): A106.

Zuccolo, L., R. Harris, D. Gunnell, et al. Height and Prostate Cancer Risk: A Large Nested Case-Controlled Study and Meta-Analysis. *Cancer Epidemiology Biomarkers & Prevention* 17, no. 9 (September 1, 2008): 2325–2326.

Sassy Kids

Almond Board of California. Almonds—At the Heart of a Healthful Diet. May 16, 2004. www.almondsarein.com.

Brand-Miller, Jennie, Johanna Burani, and Kaye Foster-Powell. *The Glucose Revolution Life Plan: Discover How to Make the Glycemic Index the Foundation for a Lifetime of Healthy Eating.* New York: Marlowe and Company, 2000.

Khan, A. M. Safdar, M. M. Ali Khan, K. N. Khattak. and R. Anderson. Cinnamon Improves Glucose and Lipids of People with Type 2 Diabetes. *Diabetes Care* 26 (December 2003): 3215–3218.

Tomaru, M., H. Takano, N. Osakabe, et al. Dietary Supplementation with Cacao Liquor Proanthocyanidins Prevents Elevation of Blood Glucose Levels in Diabetic Obese Mice. *Nutrition* 23, no. 4 (April 2007): 351–355.

Smoking Cessation

Chocolate and Your Health. *Harvard Men's Health Watch* 13, no. 7 (February 2009): 1–4.

EHealth MD. What Impact Can Diet Have on Emphysema? October 2004. www.ehealthmd.com/library/Emphysema/EMP_living.html#diet.

Greene, Bob. *Get with the Program: Getting Real About Your Weight, Health, and Emotional Well-Being.* New York: Simon & Schuster, 2002.

Heiss, Christian, Petra Kleinbongard, Andre Dejam, et al. Acute Consumption of Flavanol-Rich Cocoa and the Reversal of Endothelial Dysfunction in Smokers. *Journal of American College of Cardiology* 46, no. 7 (September 2005): 1276–1283.

Johnston, C., C. Meyer, and J. Srilakshmi. Vitamin C Elevates Red Blood Cell Glutathione in Healthy Adults. *American Journal of Clinical Nutrition* 58 (1993): 103–105.

Nicita-Mauro, V., G. Basile, G. Maltese, C. Nicita-Mauro, S. Gangemi, and C. Caruso. Smoking, Health and Ageing. *Immunity & Ageing* 5 (2008): 10.

Ozguner, F., A. Koyu, and C. Gokhan. Active Smoking Causes Oxidative Stress and Decreases Blood Melatonin Levels. *Toxicology and Industrial Health* 21, no. 10 (2005): 21–26.

Sniffles

Cold Flu Traditional Medicines. Tealand. www.tealand.com/Cold_Flu_Traditional_Medicinals.aspx.

Kulp, M., G. Mitchell, E. Borsting, et al. The Convergence Insufficiency Treatment Trial (CITT) Study Group. Effectiveness of Placebo Therapy for Maintaining Maskin in a Clinical Trial of Vergence/Accommodative Therapy. *Investigative Ophthalmology and Visual Science* 50 (2009): 2560–2566.

Lifestyle Lounge. Benefits of Peppermint. http://lifestyle.iloveindia.com/lounge/benefits-of-peppermint-6042.html.

Vitacost.com. www.vitacost.com.

Whole Foods Supplements Guide. Sources of Antioxidants. www.whole-food-supplements-guide.com/sources-of-antioxidants.html.

Spousal Discord

Braverman, E. *Younger You: Unlock the Hidden Power of Your Brain to Look and Feel 15 Years Younger.* New York: McGraw Hill, 2007.

Cousens, G., and M. Mayell. *Depression-Free for Life: A Physician's All-Natural, 5-Step Plan.* New York: HarperCollins, 2001.

Here's to Your Health and Happiness: Toasting the Benefits and Pleasures of Chocolate. Romolo Chocolates. www.romolochocolates.com.

Jacobsen, Rowan. *Chocolate Unwrapped: The Surprising Health Benefits of America's Favorite Passion.* Montpelier, VT: Invisible Cities Press, 2003.

Wolfe, David, and Shazzie. *Naked Chocolate: The Astonishing Truth About the World's Greatest Food.* San Diego: Maul Brothers, 2005.

Stress

Braverman, E. *Younger You: Unlock the Hidden Power of Your Brain to Look and Feel 15 Years Younger.* New York: McGraw Hill, 2007.

Murdock, Linda. *A Busy Cook's Guide to Spices: How to Introduce New Flavors to Everyday Meals.* Denver, CO: Bellwether Books, 2007.

Murray, Michael T. *Encyclopedia of Nutritional Supplements: The Essential Guide for Improving Your Health Naturally.* Rocklin, CA: Prima Publishing, 1996.

Warrenburg S. Effects of Fragrance on Emotions: Moods and Physiology. *Chemical Senses* 30, Suppl 1 (2005): i248–i249.

Wolfe, David, and Shazzie. *Naked Chocolate: The Astonishing Truth About the World's Greatest Food.* San Diego: Maul Brothers, 2005.

Stroke

American Stroke Association. www.StrokeAssociation.org.

Daniels, Stephen. Plasma Vitamin C Concentrations Predict Risk of Incident Stroke over 10 Y in 20649 Participants of the European Prospective Investigation into Cancer. *American Journal of Clinical Nutrition* 87 (2008): 64–69.

Das, U. Essential Fatty Acids and Their Metabolites Could Function as Endogenous HMG-CoA Reductase and ACE Enzyme Inhibitors, Anti-Arrhythmic, Anti-Hypertensive, Anti-Atherosclerotic, Anti-Inflammatory, Cytoprotective, and Cardioprotective Molecules. *Lipids in Health and Disease* 7 (2008): 37.

Soyama, Y., K. Miura, Y. Morikawa, et al. High-Density Lipoprotein Cholesterol and Risk of Stroke in Japanese Men and Women. *Stroke* 34 (2003): 863.

Sugar Overload

Atkinson, F. S., K. Foster-Powell, and J. C. Brand-Miller. International Tables of Glycemic Index and Glycemic Load Values: 2008. *Diabetes Care* 31, no. 12 (2008).

Brand-Miller, Jennie, Johanna Burani, and Kaye Foster-Powell. *The Glucose Revolution Life Plan: Discover How to Make the Glycemic Index the Foundation for a Lifetime of Healthy Eating.* New York: Marlowe and Company, 2001.

Cruise, Jorge. *8 Minutes in the Morning: A Simple Way to Shed Up to 2 Pounds a Week—Guaranteed.* New York: St. Martin's Press, 2001.

Diet Plans Web site: www.Diet-Plans.org.

Healing Daily. Web site: www.HealingDaily.com.

Jacobsen, Rowan. *Chocolate Unwrapped: The Surprising Health Benefits of America's Favorite Passion.* Montpelier, VT: Invisible Cities Press, 2003.

McCord, Holly. *Win the Sugar War: 100 Real-Life Stories of Conquering Cravings—and Pounds.* New York: St. Martin's Press, 2002.

Rosen, Kelli. The Sugar Debate. *Delicious Living*. February 1, 2008. http://deliciouslivingmag.com/food/nutrition/sugar-debate.

Vitamin Deficiency

Dean, Carolyn. *The Miracle of Magnesium: The Essential Nutrient That Works Wonders for Your Health and Energy*. New York: Ballantine Books, 2004.

Edwards, J., S. Villar, L. Fernando, C. de Oliveira, and M. Le Hyaric. Analytical Raman Spectroscopic Study of Cacao Seeds and Their Chemical Extracts. *Analytica Chimica Acta* 538 (2005):175–180.

Jacobsen, Rowan. *Chocolate Unwrapped: The Surprising Health Benefits of America's Favorite Passion*. Montpelier, VT: Invisible Cities Press, 2003.

Wolfe, David, and Shazzie. *Naked Chocolate: The Astonishing Truth About the World's Greatest Food*. San Diego: Maul Brothers, 2005.

Weight Gain

Atkinson, F. S., K. Foster-Powell, and J. C. Brand-Miller. International Tables of Glycemic Index and Glycemic Load Values: 2008. *Diabetes Care* 31, no. 12

Chocolate, Food of the Gods. *American Journal of Clinical Nutrition* 60 (1994): S1060–1067.

Ornish, Dean. *Eat More, Weigh Less: Dr. Dean Ornish's Life Choice Program for Losing Weight Safely While Eating Abundantly*. New York: HarperCollins, 1993.

Truby, H., S. Baic, A. deLooy, et al. Randomized Controlled Trial of Four Commercial Weight Loss Programs in the UK: Initial Findings from the BBC "Diet Trials." *British Medical Journal* 332 (June 2006): 1309–1314.

Wolfe, David, and Shazzie. *Naked Chocolate: The Astonishing Truth About the World's Greatest Food*. San Diego: Maul Brothers, 2005

Yoshioka, M., S. St-Pierre, and V. Drapeau. Effects of Red Pepper on Appetite and Energy Intake. *British Journal of Nutrition* 82 (1999): 115–123.

Yuan, C., L. Dey, J. Xie, and H. Aung. Gastric Effects of Galanin and Its Interaction with Leptin on Brainstem Neuronal Activity. *Journal of Pharmacology and Experimental Therapeutics* 301, no. 2 (May 2002): 488–493.

8. Chocolate and Wine Pairing

Benjamin, Barbara Bloch. *The Little Black Book of Chocolate*. NewYork: Peter Pauper Press, 2003.

Bloom, Carole. *Chocolate Lover's Cookbook for Dummies*. New York: John Wiley & Sons, 2002.

Coe, Sophie D., and Michael D. Coe. *The True History of Chocolate*. New York: Thames and Hudson, 1996.

DeSaulniers, Marcel, and Ron Manville. *I'm Dreaming of a Chocolate Christmas*. Hoboken, NJ, John Wiley & Sons, 2007.

Didio, Tony, and Amy Zavatto. *Renaissance Guide to Wine and Food Pairing*. Indianapolis, IN: Alpha Books, 2003.

Food and Wine Pairing. www.foodandwinepairing.org/food_pairing_board.html.

Hasson, Julie. *300 Best Chocolate Recipes*. Toronto, Ontario: Robert Rose, 2006.

Jefford, Andrew. *Choosing Wine*. New York: Ryland Peters & Small, 2003

Junior League of Denver, Inc. *Colorado Colore: A Palate of Tastes*. Nashville: Favorite Recipes Press, 2002.

Murdock, Linda. *A Busy Cook's Guide to Spices: How to Introduce New Flavors to Everyday Meals*. Denver, CO: Bellwether Books, 2007.

Murray, Michael T. *The Encyclopedia of Healing Foods*. New York: Atria Books, 2005.

The Pantry. Chocolate and Cocoa. Baking 911. Chocolate Basics. www.baking911.com/chocolate/basics.htm.

Raffaldini. www.raffaldini.com/grapes.shtml.

Red Wine Academy. www.redwineacademy.com/types-of-redwine-grapes.html.

Ristoraunte Amarone. www.loscabosguide.com/amarone/index.html.

Schott, Lauren, and Thomas Dhellemmes. *The Seven Sins of Chocolate*. New York: DK Publishing, 2006.

Index

About the Author

Julie Pech has embodied a passion for nutrition and health her entire life. As a longtime competitor in sports, she was always interested in nutrition for performance. She studied science and nutrition in college and earned a degree in psychology from the University of Colorado in Denver. After thirteen years in the sporting goods industry, she left to start her own company, then sold it five successful years later to follow her dream of becoming an author. Finally capitalizing on her psychology degree, she set out to prove that when you combine the mind, the body, and chocolate, something extraordinary happens.

Julie speaks up to twenty times a month to groups of all kinds about the health benefits of chocolate. She teaches chocolate and wine pairing and chocolate and tea pairing classes and travels internationally as a guest lecturer on cruise ships—speaking about chocolate, of course. She also enjoys creating new all-natural chocolates at her chocolate and coffee shop, The Chocolate Therapist, in downtown Littleton, Colorado, where the chocolates are hand-crafted in the store. The shop makes custom orders for every occasion, from private label bars to wedding favors to custom-molded chocolates and more. The chocolates are always handcrafted and all-natural. For information, e-mail info@thechocolatetherapist.com or call 303-795-7913.

A percentage of all of her book profits benefits worldwide children's programs. Julie also supports nonprofit organizations by donating a percentage of book sales to groups that host book signings. You may contact her through her Web site at www.TheChocolateTherapist.com.